Psychiatry, Subjectivity, Community

ITALIAN MODERNITIES

VOL. 15

Edited by
Pierpaolo Antonello and Robert Gordon,
University of Cambridge

PETER LANG

Oxford · Bern · Berlin · Bruxelles · Frankfurt am Main · New York · Wien

Psychiatry, Subjectivity, Community

Franco Basaglia and Biopolitics

Alvise Sforza Tarabochia

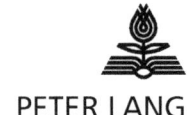

PETER LANG

Oxford · Bern · Berlin · Bruxelles · Frankfurt am Main · New York · Wien

Bibliographic information published by Die Deutsche Nationalbibliothek
Die Deutsche Nationalbibliothek lists this publication in the Deutsche
Nationalbibliografie; detailed bibliographic data is available on the Internet
at http://dnb.d-nb.de.

A catalogue record for this book is available from the British Library.

Library of Congress Control Number: 2013933468

Cover image: Franco Basaglia rams a bench against the gates of the
San Giovanni asylum in Trieste in an attempt to get the sculpture
Marco Cavallo out of the premises (1973) © Neva Gasparo.

ISSN 1662-9108
ISBN 978-3-0343-0893-9

© Peter Lang AG, International Academic Publishers, Bern 2013
Hochfeldstrasse 32, CH-3012 Bern, Switzerland
info@peterlang.com, www.peterlang.com, www.peterlang.net

All rights reserved.
All parts of this publication are protected by copyright.
Any utilisation outside the strict limits of the copyright law, without
the permission of the publisher, is forbidden and liable to prosecution.
This applies in particular to reproductions, translations, microfilming,
and storage and processing in electronic retrieval systems.

Contents

Acknowledgements — vii

Note on References — ix

Introduction — 1

CHAPTER 1
Basaglia and Psychiatry in the 1950s — 13

CHAPTER 2
The Subject and the Body — 35

CHAPTER 3
The 1960s: Challenging Psychiatry — 65

CHAPTER 4
'The Destruction of the Asylum' — 95

CHAPTER 5
Biopolitics and Psychiatry — 135

CHAPTER 6
Towards an Affirmative Biopolitical Psychiatry — 171

Bibliography — 193

Index — 213

Acknowledgements

This book would not have been possible without many exceptional people, who have helped me, in different ways, over many years.

I owe all that I have done and much more to Wissia Fiorucci who has always been there for me, emotionally and intellectually, stimulating my ideas, clarifying doubts and never letting uncertainty get in the way of creativity. No word suffices to acknowledge my parents, who have patiently and ceaselessly encouraged me on my life path.

No small thanks are due to Marco Piasentier, with whom I engaged in so many heated discussions that at least half of my ideas (if not much more) took shape while talking to him. I would also like to thank Angelos Evangelou, who has kindly helped me in my work on difficult sections.

I am much indebted to Professor Lorenzo Chiesa for all his support during the years I have worked on this project and also to Dr Francesco Capello.

I would also like to thank wholeheartedly Maureen Speller for her impressively accurate proofreading. I express my gratitude to Mario Colucci for his help in this project during its embryonic stages, and also to Giuseppe Dell'Acqua, Giovanna Gallio, Franco Rotelli and, last but certainly not least, Pier Aldo Rovatti.

Note on References

All cited works have been referenced using Harvard In-Text style. If the work is cited in its original language of publication, the year refers to the actual date of publication of the text consulted. If the citation is from a work that has been translated into either Italian or English, the year refers to the publication date of the translation.

In order to avoid confusion a different criterion has been applied to the following large collections of essays:

> Franco Basaglia, *Scritti*, ed. Franca Ongaro Basaglia, vols i–ii (Turin: Einaudi, 1981).
> Franco Basaglia, *L'utopia della realtà*, ed. Franca Ongaro Basaglia (Turin: Einaudi, 2005).

In these two cases the date in the in-text citation refers to the original publication date of the paper cited. Correspondingly, the name of the author in the bibliography is followed by the original date of publication date of the paper cited, whereas the publication date of the collection of essays is given at the end of the bibliographical reference.

Introduction

The Reform of Italian Psychiatry: Law 180/1978

On 13 May 1978, four days after Aldo Moro was executed by the Red Brigades, the Italian Parliament voted on and passed Law 180. Since then, Italy has been at the forefront of psychiatric healthcare worldwide as a result of the radical changes that Law 180 brought about: in particular, the eradication of psychiatric hospitals and the strict regulation of involuntary hospitalisation in psychiatric units. Thus, the potential lifelong incarceration of patients has been reduced to a seven-day treatment process, carried out with proper respect for their human rights. Simultaneously, Law 180 introduced a radical community approach to Italian psychiatry, based in local centres (*Centri di Salute Mentale*) and supported by the *Servizio Psichiatrico di Diagnosi e Cura* (SPDC), small (fifteen-bed) units in general hospitals, which provide acute short-term inpatient treatment. Many countries (such as France and the United Kingdom) had adopted a community approach to psychiatry before Italy, while others, most notably Brazil, are presently moving towards an 'Italian' model, i.e. a psychiatric service based exclusively on timely community intervention rather than long-term confinement. Yet, to date, globally, 63 per cent of psychiatric beds are still located in long-term facilities, only 44 per cent of the countries have structures that provide psychosocial interventions, and 67 per cent of financing is directed towards mental hospitals (WHO, 2011: 10–11). The Italian experience in psychiatry is unique, having completely abandoned the psychiatric hospital, and the World Health Organization recognises this uniqueness, in that it regards Italy as a 'punto di riferimento per le politiche planetarie di salute mentale' (Piccione, 2004: 67).

The system is not flawless, however. The first significant exception to the implementation of Law 180, the six *Ospedali Psichiatrici Giudiziari*

(OPG), which admit convicted criminals diagnosed with a mental illness, should soon be transformed as, after an inquiry led by Senator Ignazio Marino, the government has decreed the closure of the OPGs by 2013. Proposals to recreate similar structures are already emerging, but the matter is far from settled, at least at the time of writing. The OPGs account for a total of approximately 1,500 inpatients, interned in very harsh conditions. The number of inpatients is very modest compared to the 96,000 psychiatric patients hospitalised in 1968 (Ongaro Basaglia, 1987: xxiv) but is nevertheless an inconsistency within the Italian psychiatric health care system. Secondly, there is still the issue of private residential facilities, which offered, at the time of the last census (2000), 17,138 inpatient beds: three times the public provision in the SPDCs. The conditions within these private structures are difficult to monitor. Thirdly, Law 180 has been implemented at a different pace and to very different extents in individual regions. While Friuli-Venezia Giulia, the Veneto and Tuscany, for instance, have very efficient *Dipartimenti di Salute Mentale*, others, mainly because of a lack of funding, heavily rely on pre-Law 180 systems, redirecting patients to private residential facilities, enforcing physical constraint, and so on. The extent of this 'patchy' implementation, as Donnelly (1992: 81) calls it, is difficult if not impossible to assess, for few if any nationwide studies have been carried out since the approval of Law 180 (Corbellini and Jervis, 2008: 163).

It may also be because of this that numerous attempts have been made to counter these reforms in psychiatry, the latest being the *Proposta di Legge* put forward by a number of deputies of the *Lega Nord* and of the centre-right coalition on 22 April 2010, which was reproposed several times, in the form of consolidated and amended texts.[1] Most of these proposals introduced longer and stricter involuntary hospitalisations, emphasised the importance of the private sector, reintroduced semi-residential facilities

---

1 The full text of all the relevant proposals and the minutes of the Parliamentary discussions are available at this address: http://www.camera.it/cartellecomuni/leg16/documenti/progettidilegge/IFT/formEstrazione.asp?pdl=3421 [accessed 15 March 2011].

and stressed psychiatry's role in social protection. Significantly, none of the earlier proposals ever passed.

When Law 180 was approved, Italian psychiatry was still regulated by a law dating back to 1904 (*Legge 36/1904*) which, in brief, noted the social dangers represented by the mentally ill and provided for their involuntary (and potentially lifelong) internment in an asylum. Italian psychiatry was practised in abysmal conditions compared with other European countries (Ongaro Basaglia, 1987: xii). Psychotherapeutic, social and community approaches, in spite of their progress abroad, were not introduced into Italian psychiatry – known as *freniatria* (from the Ancient Greek *phren*, which meant mind or brain) precisely to avoid any reference to what was regarded as an overtly 'spiritual' notion, that of 'psyche' (Donnelly, 1992: 30) – until the years leading up to 1978. The main response to the problem of mental illness before this date amounted to internment in the asylum and to therapeutic approaches with very dubious, if not entirely pathogenic, results, such as shock therapies and psychosurgery. Among those 'alternative' psychiatrists who fought against this backward scenario and eventually succeeded in persuading Italian psychiatry to catch up with ideas of progress in community and social approaches that were being implemented abroad, Franco Basaglia is certainly the best remembered. It was thanks to Basaglia's political activism that the general population was made aware of the backwardness of Italian psychiatry and that, eventually, this problem came to the attention of the psychiatrist and Christian Democrat Senator, Bruno Orsini, who formulated Law 180 and pushed for its approval in the Italian Parliament. Although Basaglia could count on a team of prominent collaborators and followers in his everyday psychiatric practice – first among them, his wife, Franca Ongaro – and while his political activism was backed by the group *Psichiatria Democratica*, which he co-founded in 1973, it is mainly thanks to his unceasing reforms in the asylums of which he was director and to his public propaganda campaigns that a wide spectrum of the population developed an awareness of psychiatric issues and the Italian Parliament recognised the necessity of reforming psychiatry through the law.

Franco Basaglia and His Legacy

After graduating in paediatric neurobiology at the University of Padua, specialising in *malattie nervose e mentali* and working for a university clinic, Franco Basaglia (Venice, 1924–80) directed three asylums: first Gorizia (1961–69), then Colorno (1969–71) and, finally, Trieste (1971–79). In Gorizia, Basaglia began to experiment with possible alternatives to the harsh institutional conditions that he witnessed there. He abolished the wearing of white coats to lessen the perceived distance between the doctor and the patient, abandoned all forms of physical restriction, such as straitjackets and cage-beds, and finally unlocked the wards of the asylum. It was during his years in Gorizia that he developed the idea that the main obstacle to the advancement of a more 'humane' form of psychiatry was the asylum itself: even if it was possible to 'humanise' the psychiatric hospital, as had already been done in many European countries, its persistence would still mean that psychiatry might only respond to social/moral demands rather than to actual medical needs. As long as the asylum, albeit humanised, was allowed to stand, psychiatry would be entrusted with the separation of deviant individuals, the insane, and so on, from 'healthy' society.

In 1964, Basaglia declared his intentions: 'la distruzione del manicomio è un fatto urgentemente necessario, se non semplicemente ovvio' (Basaglia, 1964a: 19). The administration of the province of Gorizia was too conservative to permit Basaglia and his team to implement the radical reforms that would lead to the demise of the psychiatric hospital and Basaglia moved first to Colorno and then to Trieste. Here, Basaglia not only implemented all the reforms he had carried out in Gorizia, he also began to prepare the 'community' for the closure of the asylum.

This preparation involved various initiatives, most notably a campaign to raise the awareness of the Triestine population with respect to psychiatric health care issues. Among various examples, we might mention a parade through the city organised by the inmates and the psychiatric workers of the asylum, led by the iconic blue papier-mâché horse, Marco Cavallo (23 March 1973); the flight organised for the inmates by Alitalia on 16 September 1975 and, finally, the renting of a holiday house, *Villa Fulcis*, in Belluno (1975).

These initiatives played a key role in raising public awareness and finally bring the issue of psychiatric health care in Parliament, where Basaglia's pioneering work was transformed into Law 180. Basaglia was to die only two years later, leaving the actual implementation of the law, the gradual closure of all Italian asylums and the relocation of psychiatric health care to community centres, in the hands of his followers.

What happened in the next thirty years is difficult to reconstruct in brief, mainly because of the scarcity of consistent censuses and statistical data concerning psychiatric health care in Italy. What is quite clear is that psychiatry in Italy has found itself in the difficult situation of having to reconcile a biomedical approach – the rise of the 'second biological psychiatry' (Shorter, 1997: 239) – with a radically deinstitutionalised community approach based on the Basaglian legacy. A third position, the psychotherapeutic one, is scarcely represented in public psychiatric health care (although it is an important player in the *private* sector). Behind these two or three dominant tendencies there continues to be a strong political and social pressure on psychiatrists to 'protect' society from the hazards of mental illness, a tendency that, as Basaglia foresaw in 1976, is emphasised in times of economic crisis, when the criteria for what constitutes normality usually narrow (Basaglia, 1976: 386). To date, a synthesis between the biomedical approach, Basaglia's legacy and socio-political pressure has proved difficult, if not impossible.

Towards a Possible Affirmative Biopolitics

Pierangelo Di Vittorio (2006: 73) does not hesitate to call 'biopolitical' the psychiatry that arose after the dismantling of the asylum. According to Di Vittorio, 'biopolitical' psychiatry responds, as much as the old 'institutional' psychiatry of the asylum, to the socio-political needs of identifying, preventing and dealing with the social and material dangers allegedly represented by the mentally sick person, and the need to do so primarily in organic terms, by focusing on the neurobiological and biochemical mechanisms of mental illness. The reform and, with it, the work of deinstitutionalisation that Basaglia initiated – that is to say, the overcoming of any institutional logic in psychiatry, or in Piccione's words (2004: 13), the 'percorso di critica teorico-pratica all'interno dell'apparato istituzionale psichiatrico, inteso come luogo, disciplina, procedure, norme, ecc.' – can be deemed successful so far as the demise of the asylum and institutional psychiatry is concerned. Yet, they might also have contributed to the rise of a different form of psychiatry, which answers, as much as the old institutional counterpart, a social and political mandate rather than being a medical science: Di Vittorio's 'biopolitical psychiatry'.

In calling it 'biopolitical', Di Vittorio is drawing on Michel Foucault's definition of 'biopolitics', a notion that has recently conquered 'un ruolo di primo piano nel dibattito teorico internazionale' (Esposito, 2005: 158). Although it is a term that dates back to at least the beginning of the twentieth century, the most influential formulation of biopolitics was certainly Foucault's, who defined it, together with the ambiguously connected notion of 'biopower', as the power 'to foster life or disallow it to the point of death' (Foucault, 1998: 138). In brief, Foucault defines 'biopolitics' as a tendency, which emerged in the late eighteenth century but gained unprecedented importance with the rise of neoliberalism in the 1930s, to rationalise the art of governing, on the one hand, while on the other to govern the very biological lives of the people. In other words, biopolitics marks a tendency to co-implicate life and politics. Yet Foucault's conceptualisation of biopolitics is profoundly ambiguous, and all those who dwell on the concept notice it without fail. If biopolitics can foster, promote, manage and optimise life, by means of the same direct co-implication between politics and life, it can also disallow and limit it, to the point of destroying the very life that it set forth to foster: biopolitics can drift into thanatopolitics.

This is not the only point that Foucault leaves blurred. Another issue is the evolution of power. In Foucault's model, at least two paradigms of power preceded biopolitics and were, to a certain extent, superseded by it: sovereignty and disciplinary power. Sovereignty establishes an asymmetrical relationship between the ruler and the subjects, and is imposed through a 'subtraction': the sovereign limits the freedom of the multitude by imposing taxes, levies, and so on (Foucault, 2006b: 42–46). Disciplinary power is rather different: it is a direct exertion of power that invests the very bodies of the subjects; it is exerted by means of exercises, training and subtle techniques that encourage the subject to yield to power by making him/her introject it. The ultimate aim of disciplinary power is to remove the space in which power is exerted: individuals discipline themselves. Disciplinary power spreads during the nineteenth century, although its shape is already recognisable in certain medieval monastic communities. Characteristic of disciplinary power is its exertion within dedicated institutions: the barracks, the school, the prison and, case in point, the old mental hospital, the asylum (Foucault, 1991: 145*ff*).

While at times Foucault seems to suggest that biopolitics replaces sovereignty, establishing clear-cut dichotomies is difficult, to the point that Agamben (2005) affirms that, all things considered, sovereignty in general, since at least Ancient Rome, has been biopolitical. The issue is even more complicated when it comes to distinguishing between discipline and biopolitics: according to Foucault (2003b: 242), the latter exploits techniques and apparatuses of the former; it embeds them and systematises their application. Disciplinary power is localised, for instance, inside institutions, whereas biopolitics is widespread and it entails a rational exertion of political power on the entire population. In order to exploit disciplinary techniques to reach the entirety of the population, biopolitics makes use of ancillary specialistic bodies of knowledge such as epidemiology or statistics. For instance, if exercises and teachings to improve personal hygiene (in a school, for example) might be considered 'disciplinary', their systematisation, based on cost-benefit studies, in turn based on epidemiological surveys demonstrating that increased personal hygiene reduces the risk of spreading of certain diseases, supported by nationwide campaigns of awareness, could be regarded as 'biopolitical'.

In his 1973–74 course at the *Collège de France* entitled *Le Pouvoir psychiatrique*, Foucault (2006b) uses the nineteenth-century asylum and its 'institutional' psychiatry as the perfect example of disciplinary power. Upon admission to the asylum inmates are required to forfeit their identity and identify completely with the institution, which will dictate every single aspect of their lives until discharge or death. Inmates are reduced to docile individuals whose very bodies are subjected to the allegedly therapeutic physical treatments, such as shock therapies and sedative cocktails, and are constrained in numerous ways (e.g. handcuffs, straitjackets, cage-beds). Inpatients would be considered as healed – if this ever happened – only when they were able to discipline themselves.

Franco Basaglia faced a very similar scenario. In the 1950s, psychiatry in Italy had been lagging behind the rest of Europe: social and community interventions were hardly considered and mental disorder was addressed almost exclusively in terms of a strongly institutionalised biological psychiatry, which was grounded in the notion that mental illness was an organic disease that could be treated with physical 'therapies' in the isolation of the asylum. Apart from the mental hospital, those suffering from a mental disorder could rely on university and private clinics, but only if they could afford the high fees. For the poor, the indigent and social deviants, only the public asylum was available. Hence, Basaglia came to understand the mental hospital as the place where 'sane' – bourgeois – society locked away its contradictions and its obscene byproducts (Basaglia, 1975a: 239). Humanising the management and everyday praxis in the mental hospital – for instance, by abolishing physical constraint, opening the wards, adopting limited open-door solutions, etc. – was no use: albeit humane, the mental hospital would still be the place where society could 'dump' its deviants (Basaglia, 1964a: 18*ff*). Its purpose would still be 'disciplinary': inpatients would be discharged when they became 'collaborative', 'docile', 'accustomed to social norms', and so on (Basaglia, 1965c: 287). The demise of the asylum was the only possibility to overcome the disciplinary aspect of psychiatry and envision a new psychiatry: not a better, more efficient, more humane or more effective medical science for the treatment of mental illness, but a psychiatry that could be at the service of those suffering from a mental disorder instead of (bourgeois) society.

From this perspective, the reform was successful: public mental health care has been completely diverted to community centres, which often work on a 24/7 open-door basis; involuntary treatment lasts as little as seven days and can only be enforced if it benefits the patient and not because he/she poses a threat to society. If one excludes the cases of 'neo-manicomialità' (Piccione, 2004: 118), that mark a return to a disciplinary form of psychiatry even in the community centres and show that the work of deinstitutionalisation is never completely finished, 'disciplinary psychiatry' or, at least, the disciplinary character of a certain psychiatry, was overcome.

However, not unlike biopolitics in general according to Foucault, 'biopolitical psychiatry' seems to have risen from the ashes of 'disciplinary psychiatry'. Many examples could clarify what is meant by 'biopolitical psychiatry': childhood screenings to diagnose, treat and prevent mental disorders as early in life as possible; the introduction of psychiatric interventions in primary-care contexts; a heightened attention towards epidemiological studies concerning mental disorders; the widespread psychiatrisation of normal phases of life (such as adolescence or old age) or states (such as bereavement, situational stress, etc.); their consequent medicalisation (especially in terms of pharmacological intervention); and the list could continue. Instead of being practised within the enclosed walls of the institution, psychiatry now seems to directly influence daily life. And it also seems to continue serving socio-political and moral mandates rather than therapeutic ones: preventing and dealing with anti-social behaviour, helping individuals cope with difficult situations and thus enable them to remain productive, and so on.

Basaglia was certainly aware of this possible outcome of the work of deinstitutionalisation and, in 1979, during one of the conferences he delivered in Brazil (the proceedings of which were published as *Conferenze Brasiliane*, 2000), he reiterated his view that widespread medicalisation and psychiatrisation of everyday life are a 'nuovo manicomio' against which we must act (Basaglia, 2000: 181). However, Basaglia died one year later and was thus unable to witness the rise of 'biopolitical psychiatry'.

Basaglia's work should not be regarded as obsolete because of this, as if the revolutionary potential of his writings had exhausted itself after successfully bringing about the demise of the asylum. Nor should Basaglia's work be read *only* as an instrument with which to fight against the last remaining instances of 'disciplinary psychiatry', in Italy and abroad. I strongly believe that Basaglia's work can and should be reread in the light of biopolitics and this book is the result of this belief. Yet, at the same time, I do not think that Basaglia should be reread in the light of biopolitics in order to wage war against 'biopolitical psychiatry', which is what many thinkers of the Basaglian legacy – chiefly among them Colucci and Di Vittorio – seem to suggest. And this is mainly because I believe that biopolitics itself must still be read in the light of the original ambiguity with which Foucault presented it: as much as biopolitics can foster life, it can also disallow it. That these two views rest on the same original co-implication of life and politics means that envisioning an affirmative biopolitics, capable of preventing biopolitics itself from drifting into thanatopolitics, is all the more urgent. To understand whether this will prove possible in the context of psychiatry, and whether the premises of such a hypothetical and maybe utopian 'affirmative biopolitical psychiatry' can be traced back to Basaglia, is the challenge of this book.

* * *

The first chapter is dedicated to contextualising the early work of Franco Basaglia. To do so, I present a summary intellectual biography of Basaglia, along with an overview of the state of psychiatry worldwide and especially in Italy, when he began to practise as a physician in 1953. In those years, few alternatives were available to mainstream biological and institutional psychiatry, and one of the most influential to Basaglia was so-called phenomenological psychiatry, which I introduce in this chapter with particular attention to the works of Karl Jaspers and Ludwig Binswanger.

The second chapter is initially devoted to analysing some of Basaglia's first written works, namely 'Il mondo dell'incomprensibile schizofrenico' (1953) and 'Su alcuni aspetti della moderna psicoterapia: analisi fenomenologica dell'incontro' (1954), in which I highlight the influence of phenomenological psychiatry. The focus then moves to different writings by Basaglia from the decade covering 1957–67, in which I retrieve and examine the fundamental tripartite relationship between the notions of 'subject', 'body' and 'other'.

The writings from between 1957 and 1967, belong to an era of great tumult in psychiatry: the 1960s and 1970s. Psychiatrists such as R.D. Laing, David Cooper, the recently deceased Thomas Szasz, Frantz Fanon and others, as well as Basaglia himself, began to question psychiatry on sociopolitical rather than medical grounds, earning the much contested and often rejected label of 'anti-psychiatrists'. The first part of Chpater 3 is dedicated to a summarising overview of 'anti-psychiatry'. In the second part, I focus more closely on one of the most influential thinkers of this period, who, as has already been suggested, kindled the challenging of psychiatry during the 1960s and 1970s; namely, Michel Foucault. The analysis begins with his *Folie et Déraison* and concludes with the definition of 'disciplinary power' in relation to psychiatry in the two courses at the *Collège de France*, *Le Pouvoir psychiatrique* and *Les Anormaux*.

In Chapter 4, the focus returns to Basaglia, in order to present the main tenets that guided his reforming praxis in the three asylums he directed: Gorizia, Colorno and finally Trieste. Two are the central points of this analysis: his clinical approach – based on his influential notion of 'bracketing mental illness'; that is to say, disregarding the patients' diagnoses and understanding them in the wider social and political context that excluded them in the first place – and his 'political activism', grounded in the comparison between reforming psychiatrists and *engagé* intellectuals. In doing so, I highlight the central importance that Basaglia gave to the notions of 'social contradiction' and utopia. In concluding this chapter, Law 180 and Basaglia's own comments on and criticisms of the law are discussed.

Law 180 has been subject of many criticisms, and among them the fact that it may have facilitated the rise of so-called 'biopolitical psychiatry'. In Chapter 5 this notion is presented with the aim of criticising the exclusively negative aura that has been ascribed to it hitherto. In the first part of the chapter distinctions are drawn between the positive and negative aspects of 'biopolitics', as understood by Foucault. In the second, having applied this 'tension' to the context of psychiatry, I give a schematic overview of how this medical science is practised today, relying on the most recent studies and surveys. I believe this helps to delineate what some authors understand as 'biopolitical psychiatry' or at least psychiatry as it is practised in the era of biopolitics.

The book concludes with Chapter 6, where I recover from Basaglia's own work the embryonic conception of a possible 'affirmative' connotation of 'biopolitical psychiatry'. The main theoretical framework for this chapter is the work of the Italian philosopher Roberto Esposito, who has recognised the ambiguities left by Foucault himself in defining biopolitics and hypothesised the possibility of an affirmative biopolitics capable of preventing the contrary drift into forms of thanatopolitics.

CHAPTER 1

Basaglia and Psychiatry in the 1950s

Introduction

The groundbreaking extent of Law 180 and the innovative transformations that Basaglia's work brought about cannot be fully understood if we abstract them from the context of how psychiatry was practised in Italy in the 1950s, the years when Basaglia concluded his medical studies and began practising as a psychiatrist in Giovanni Battista Belloni's university clinic in Padua. After presenting a short intellectual biography of Franco Basaglia, this chapter therefore features an introductory overview of psychiatry, beginning with its situation in the first half of the twentieth century. The general concerns of the relatively young medical specialty of psychiatry are presented, with particular attention to aetiological theories, diagnostic criteria and available treatments. I then give a more detailed picture of how psychiatry was practised in Italy, discussing also the principal laws that regulated the administration of psychiatric treatments and admission to the main structure in which psychiatry was practised, at least until the 1978 reform: the psychiatric hospital, i.e. the asylum, the public *manicomio*.

In Italy, when Basaglia became a psychiatrist, the mainstream doctrine in psychiatry was biological and institutional. In brief, on the one hand, mental illness was believed to be a disease like any other, with an organic origin (be it in the brain, in the nerves or in the endocrine system) and therefore requiring an appropriate physical treatment (shock therapies, psychosurgery, and so on). On the other hand, there was a deeply rooted belief that institutionalisation – the involuntary prolonged hospitalisation of mental patients – was beneficial in itself, hence the predominance of asylum-centred treatments in Italy in contrast to the rest of Europe, where, at least after World War II, numerous experiments in social, community and rehabilitative approaches to psychiatry were producing promising results.[1] There were a few alternatives to this perspective, most notably an approach hardly known in Italy until Basaglia himself among others introduced it: so-called 'phenomenological' or 'existential' psychiatry, a multifaceted approach grounded more in a philosophical study of the existence of the human being than in a medical study of the anatomical body of the mental patient. I briefly present this current in psychiatry, concluding this chapter with the introduction of the central notions and main representatives of phenomenological psychiatry. Particular attention is given to Jaspers' phenomenological psychopathology and Binswanger's introduction of existentialist concerns in his *Daseinsanalyse*, two crucial steps in the definition of the multifaceted phenomeno-existentialist approach in psychiatry that greatly influenced Basaglia's early work.

A Brief Intellectual Biography of Franco Basaglia

Franco Basaglia was born on 11 March 1924 in Venice, where he spent most of his childhood. In 1943, when Northern Italy was under the Nazi-Fascist regime, he began his studies at the University of Padua. It was here that the young Basaglia became a member of a student antifascist group and, following subversive activities, was arrested by Fascist squads; Basaglia's first experience of a 'total institution' (Goffman, 2007), the prison, lasted six months. Graduating in 1949 in *medicina e chirurgia*, having defended a

---

[1] For instance, in France Georges Daumézon and Philippe Koechlin (1952) began to implement the so-called *psychoterápie institutionelle*; that is, they introduced a psychoanalytical approach in psychiatric health care. In the United Kingdom, Bion and Rickman began to experiment with several kinds of social approaches (see Mills and Harrison, 2007). These converged in Maxwell Jones's therapeutic community, a practice that Basaglia implemented later in Gorizia's asylum.

thesis on paediatric neurobiology, Basaglia specialised in *malattie nervose e mentali*. In 1953, he joined Giovanni Battista Belloni's *Clinica di malattie nervose e mentali*, a university clinic in Padua, where he worked until 1961. In the same year he married Franca Ongaro, initially a creative writer, with whom he shared his lifelong commitment to the reform of psychiatric health care. Franca Ongaro was a central figure in the reform carried out by Basaglia and his team: she translated into Italian a number of key texts, such as Goffman's *Asylums* in 1969; with her husband she co-wrote and co-edited several essays and books, including *Che cos'è la psichiatria?* in 1967 and *L'istituzione negata* in 1968. After Basaglia's death, she continued his legacy, served as a Senator from 1984 to 1991, and actively contributed to the application and implementation of Law 180, the law that radically reformed psychiatric health care in Italy.

Franca Ongaro also edited Basaglia's *Scritti*, a two-volume selection of his papers, published posthumously in 1981, the key work for understanding Basaglia's biopolitics and much else in his thought. In the introduction to the first volume of his writings (Basaglia, 1981b: xix–xliv), Basaglia's work is divided into four different phases. The first, 'psychopathological', phase consists of his first six essays, and is purely scientific: the strictly biological orientation of the clinic in which he worked heavily influenced Basaglia's early papers. In his own words:

> la prima fase può essere ritenuta il segno del primo contatto con la cultura psichiatrica e dell'adattamento pedissequo ai parametri di una scienza che presenta l'oggetto e gli strumenti della sua analisi come dati fissi e indiscutibili. (Basaglia, 1981a: xix)

The second phase marks Basaglia's first attempts to address general human problems instead of specific scientific issues. He considered it as a phase dedicated to studying 'l'uomo nella sua globalità' (Basaglia, 1981a: xx). During this phase the influence of phenomenological psychiatry and *Daseinsanalyse* becomes clear; the person suffering from mental illness is no longer approached in a strictly medical way as the aim is rather to understand the patient's existence:

la fenomenologia esistenziale poteva essere, dunque, un primo strumento di smascheramento del terreno ideologico su cui la scienza si fonda. (Basaglia, 1981a: xx)[2]

Basaglia developed his interests in philosophy during his years in Belloni's clinic. Dissatisfied with the conduction of psychiatry within the university, Basaglia felt the need to move into the asylum, which psychiatrists considered to be a second-best choice and a dead end in one's career. In 1961, Gorizia's asylum appointed Basaglia as its director. Here he began his work of deinstitutionalisation, applying several reforms to the psychiatric hospital and gradually opening up its wards. It was in Gorizia that Basaglia developed his ambition of dismantling the asylum by using the law.

During the final years of his experience in Gorizia, which he left in 1969, Basaglia began the third phase of his work, which he defined as 'negazione istituzionale'. He believed this to be the most important stage in reforming psychiatric health care. In this phase, Basaglia set out to 'unmask' the scientific ideology that, in his opinion, biological and institutional psychiatry represented. Yet this stance almost naturally led him to the idea that the asylum, the very psychiatric institution itself, should be dismantled. After analysing what happens to the inmate inside the institution, Basaglia insisted on the importance of social and structural changes, such as abolishing physical constraints (e.g. straitjackets, cage-beds, etc.) and shock therapies (e.g. electroshock) in favour of a social and communicative approach (e.g. Jones's 'therapeutic community').[3] It was time to 'mettere tra parentesi la malattia mentale' (Basaglia, 1981a: xxii), an expression that owes much

---

2   On this point, it is interesting to note the words of Benedetto Saraceno, the director of psychiatric health care for World Health Organization at the time of writing. Saraceno recognised the importance of Basaglia's early thought, and the influence it had on his later political activism, on the occasion of an international conference on Basaglia's legacy (*Comunicare il pensiero, il lavoro e l'eredità di Franco Basaglia nel mondo*, Trieste, Italy, April 2008). Saraceno claims that Basaglia is generally unknown in the Anglo-Saxon world mostly because of a resistance towards phenomenology as a philosophy.

3   Jones's therapeutic community is a participative and group-based approach to the treatment of mental illness. It is best applied in residential and long-stay facilities, where patients meet with trained nurses and psychiatrists to discuss their condition

to Husserlian phenomenology, as I shall discuss later. During this phase of his work, Basaglia discovered how the institution is an organ of social control rather than a means of achieving and preserving mental health.

In 1969, Basaglia moved to Colorno (Parma), where he stayed for two years, but was unable to enforce a proper reform of the institution.[4] In 1971 he became the director of the Trieste asylum where he stayed until 1979, a year after Law 180 was approved. The fourth and last phase of his work was the actual dismantling of the institution, from the internal reforms carried out in the asylum at Trieste to the enforcement and implementation of Law 180. This journey is documented in the last phase of Basaglia's writings. After the approval of Law 180, and after beginning to implement it in Trieste, he moved to Rome, where he was entrusted with the reconfiguration of Lazio's psychiatric health care under the terms of Law 180. He died soon after this appointment, on 29 August 1980.

Psychiatry in the First Half of the Twentieth Century

In 1953 Basaglia became a practising psychiatrist in a university clinic, a space which was physically and conceptually very distant from the *manicomio* he would later have to face. In commenting on his early years as a

---

      and recreate, in miniature, the social structure of the world outside of the asylum. See Chapter 2.

4   So far, scholars have largely neglected these two years of Basaglia's career. Recently, Giovanna Gallio edited a special issue of the journal *aut aut*, where she collected, reconstructed and commented on the minutes of several meetings between Basaglia and the staff of Colorno hospital (Gallio, 2009b). According to Gallio (2009a: 52) the minutes of the meetings enable the reader to rediscover the 'spazio di emergenza dei fatti e dei materiali di lavoro che più contano' and it is undeniable that this collection has a profound historical value in that it unravels this scarcely studied period of Basaglia's life, although it lacks a studied contextualization in Basaglia's career as a whole.

physician, Basaglia remembered that, at that time, Italian psychiatry was divided into two branches. On the one hand, there was the so-called 'piccola psichiatria', where 'i grandi psichiatri erano cresciuti' (Basaglia, 1973: 210): it was the psychiatry practised in the university clinic, that accepted only cases of alleged great scientific interest; on the other hand, there was the 'grande psichiatria, dove solo i piccoli psichiatri lavoravano – quelli che non avevano trovato migliori allocazioni' (Basaglia, 1973: 210): this was the reality of the asylum. Basaglia argued that, ultimately, the destiny of mentally ill patients depended on their financial condition: only those who could afford the high fees would be admitted to a university clinic.

Yet the psychiatry that Basaglia encountered in 1953 was not only split between the university and the asylum; it was also, as a medical specialty, in a state that Shorter (1997: 298) does not hesitate to define as 'chaos'. Although dominant trends can be identified, there was very little consensus among psychiatrists on several aspects of the discipline. To begin with, there were different theories concerning the aetiopathogenesis of mental illness in general and of specific psychiatric diseases in particular. If one excludes diseases with psychiatric symptoms that have an ascertained organic cause (such as neurosyphilis, which is caused by an infection), theories on the aetiology of psychiatric disorders were either biological (mental illness as brain dysfunction, chemical imbalance, endocrine imbalance, genetic and hereditary trait, brain lesion, neuronal issues, etc.), psychogenetic/psychodynamic (Freudian psychoanalysis, Binswanger's *Daseinanalyse*, etc.) or social (family environment as pathogenetic, etc.). During the first half of the twentieth century the biological hypothesis, although difficult if not impossible to demonstrate with the instruments available, had the most supporters, followed by the psychoanalytical one. The social hypothesis emerged mostly in Britain after World War II, and gained momentum during the so-called anti-psychiatric movements of the 1960s and 1970s. Few researchers attempted a synthesis between these aspects, which were convincingly integrated into the 'biopsychosocial' model only in 1977, thanks to the work of George L. Engel.

Understandably enough, diagnosing a mental illness was as difficult as establishing its aetiology. Neuroscientific methods of medical examination were still in development and could be applied almost exclusively in an anatomo-pathological setting (i.e. during autopsies). Therefore an organic diagnosis of mental illness was impossible – and still is – except in cases of evident traumatic brain lesion. The predominance of psychoses with no evident organic roots (the so-called 'functional' psychoses) brought about the need for a systematic albeit non-organic way to study, classify and thus recognise and diagnose mental illnesses. It is with this need in mind that the German psychiatrist Emil Kraepelin (1856–1926) created a monumental nosology; that is to say, a systematic study and classification of psychiatric syndromes, by grouping observable psychiatric symptoms into patterns, depending on how often different symptoms could be observed together, their intensity, course, and so on. His method was symptomatic and clinical: his interest was the definition of diagnostic criteria and subsequent prognoses, not the study of the aetiopathogenesis of mental illness. The sixth edition of his *Textbook of Psychiatry*, published in 1899, established such an enduring paradigm that the American Psychiatric Association used it as the foundation of the first Diagnostic–Statistic Manual (DSM–I) in 1952. However, the Kraepelinian nosology was not universally accepted and was challenged by different approaches: the psychoanalytical one and Jaspers' phenomenological psychopathology, to cite but two.

However, the main problem of psychiatry was the treatment of mental illness. The therapeutic scenario was dominated by 'shock therapies', which literally consisted of traumatising patients in various ways, such as inducing hypoglycaemic comas with insulin overdoses, inoculating them with malaria-infected blood, submerging the patient in freezing water, inducing epileptic crises through various means, such as injecting elevated doses of the cardiac stimulant Cardiazol. In 1938, an Italian neurologist, Ugo Cerletti, invented the most successful of shock therapies: electro-convulsive therapy (ECT) or electroshock, which consisted of delivering a controlled electric shock to the patient until it induced an epileptic crisis (Shorter, 1997: 208–24). This therapy is still practised today in several countries, raising an ongoing debate about its effectiveness and on the bio-ethical implications of its use.⁵ With regard to pharmacology, the use of drugs was limited to alkaloids (such as morphine), bromides and barbiturates, which could temporarily relieve psychiatric symptoms but with notable drawbacks, such as addiction, high toxicity and severe side effects. The first proper neuroleptic drug – an antihistamine named chlorpromazine, capable of inducing long-lasting recovery from psychiatric symptoms with reduced side effects – was discovered only in 1952 (Shorter, 1997: 246–55).⁶ Finally, the last resort with regard to physical therapies was psychosurgery; for instance, Fiamberti's transorbital prefrontal leucotomy, later and elsewhere nicknamed 'ice-pick' lobotomy due to its ease of application. Fiamberti's method consisted of inserting a surgical pick under the arch of the eyebrows, easily reaching into the brain and severing the frontal connection between its lobes (Armocida, 2007).⁷ Basically, the only outcome of psychosurgery was to render the patient permanently docile and quiet.

---

5   A recent paper published on the topic, 'The Effectiveness of Electroconvulsive Therapy: A Literature Review' by Read and Bentall (2010), shows that to date no study has demonstrated unquestionable positive outcomes from the use of ECT (electro-convulsive therapy).

6   Neuroleptic drugs (from the Ancient Greek 'νεῦρον', which nowadays refers to nerves, and 'λαμβάνω', which means 'to take hold of') are better known today as 'anti-psychotic drugs'. These drugs are used to counter the symptoms and effect of different psychotic and neurotic states, from schizophrenia to depression. Mild 'anti-psychotic drugs' are also used for minor ailments, such as insomnia or anxious states. Chlorpromazine was first used as a powerful anaesthetic. At a later stage, pharmacists discovered that, taken in a limited dosage, chlorpromazine had a very strong tranquillising effect, to the point that it was referred to as 'chemical lobotomy'.

7   Psychosurgery was first practised experimentally on humans in 1935 by the Nobel Prize winner Egas Moniz at the University of Lisbon. Psychosurgery is the general term encompassing several different procedures of lobotomy, which consist of severing different connections between brain tissues in order to regulate or suppress emotional reaction in the patient. Psychosurgery flourished with the introduction of the ice-pick lobotomy, which could be practised under local anaesthesia and left no visible scars. Other, less invasive kinds of lobotomy are still practised today (though rarely) in different countries (such as the United States, Finland, Sweden, United Kingdom, etc.), with debatable results.

Regarding non-physical treatments there was ergo-therapy, theorised for the first time by Hermann Simon, a German psychiatrist who had discovered that the symptoms of catatonic patients improved to the point of disappearing when the patient was forced to work for the institution. Psychiatrists often relied also on clinotherapy and rest treatment, which consisted of forcing (to varying degrees) the patient to stay in bed, whether by means of strong sedative cocktails, physical restraint or simple persuasion. Psychotherapy, especially psychoanalysis, was used in psychiatric clinical practice but not much in the context of the psychiatric hospital, where the higher number of patients made it difficult to achieve the one-to-one setting required for this approach. Finally, the most widespread treatment for psychiatric illnesses was institutionalisation itself as, since Battie theorised it in 1758, it had been believed that separating mental patients from their *milieu* and forcing them into the controlled environment of the asylum was therapeutic in itself.

To conclude, it is possible to identify at least three trends in the psychiatric approaches of the time: the dominant biological paradigm, which Basaglia called *organicismo*, psychodynamic trends and social trends. However, the dominant biological paradigm had an inconsistent approach. The organic hypothesis concerning the aetiopathogenesis of mental illness was widely accepted but it did not find a direct equivalent in terms of nosology and diagnosis: mental illness was classified and diagnosed in pseudo-statistical terms and not in terms of underlying organic causes. Similarly, treatment was physical – meaning that it targeted organic processes such as brain chemistry, convulsive reactions and so forth – but it did not target the alleged organic causes of mental illness, which were only hypothesised. What is more, there was a general consensus in the mainstream that, first and foremost, for various reasons a psychiatric patient had to be treated in the isolation of the asylum or in private clinical practice.

Psychiatry in Italy

The inconsistent approach to psychiatry decribed in the previous section was the mainstream doctrine, followed perhaps by psychoanalytically oriented approaches. However, the international community of psychiatric practice was at least debating the aforementioned different trends. In Italy prior to the 1950s, on the contrary, there was little debate and Italian psychiatry was clearly lagging behind its neighbours, as Lovell and Scheper-Hughes (1987: 9) aptly note. The branch of medicine dedicated to the study and cure of mental illness had been known as *'freniatria'* until 1931, when the *Società Italiana di Freniatria* changed its name to the *Società Italiana di Psichiatria*.[8] '*Freniatria*' had been chosen precisely to avoid any reference to psychology and its root 'psych-'. As Donnelly (1992: 30) remarks, drawing on De Peri (1984), 'psyche connoted the spirit' while the root 'fren-', 'mind' or 'brain' in Ancient Greek, suggested a closer connection with the alleged organic aetiology of mental illnesses. A few psychiatrists, most notably Weiss and Levi-Bianchini, attempted to introduce Freudian psychoanalysis but with very little support from the community of practice (Canosa, 1980: 154). This 'narrow, materialistic, and anti-spiritual foundation' (Donnelly, 1992: 28) of *freniatria* was confirmed with Giovanni Gentile's 1923 reform of the educational system which, among many other changes, excluded psychology from the faculty of medicine and conflated neurology and psychiatry in the curriculum of the *clinica delle malattie nervose e mentali*.

Along with its quasi-exclusive biological approach, Italian *freniatria* was strongly 'custodialistic', in that it stressed the importance of protecting society from the mental 'aliens', much more than did its international counterparts, and did so well into the twentieth century (at least until Mariotti's provisional law in 1968, to which I will return later). Arguably, Law 36, *Disposizioni sui manicomi e gli alienati*, hurriedly passed in 1904,[9] and a number of articles from the Fascist 'Codice Rocco' (1930) ratified the role of the alienist as the 'guardian' of society against the threat represented by madmen. Law 36 established that 'debbono essere custodite e curate nei manicomi le persone affette per qualunque causa da alienazione mentale, quando siano pericolose a se' o agli altri e riescano di pubblico scandalo'

---

8   The English equivalent, though rarely used, is 'phreniatry' or 'phreniatria'.
9   Legge 36/1904, published in *Gazzetta Ufficiale*, n. 43, 22 Febbraio 1904.

(*art. 1*). The law therefore established that asylums were to cure mentally ill patients but also to hold in custody those who were a danger to society. The law also established that admission to the asylum was to be requested by relatives, wardens or 'chiunque altro, negli interessi dell'infermo o della società' (*art. 2*), whereas discharge depended on the tribunal's or the asylum director's decision (*art. 3*). It was the latter who had full authority in the asylum (*art. 4*), and ultimate control over psychiatric hospitals was regulated by the Minister of Internal Affairs (*art. 5*). In brief, one could be committed to the asylum by proscription on the grounds of allegedly being dangerous. The logical consequence was that the direction of the asylum and, ultimately, the fate of inmates depended on judicial rather than medical decisions.

The 1930 penal code, the so-called 'Codice Rocco', strengthened the link between psychiatric and judicial apparatuses in that, among other changes, it established that all patients involuntarily committed to a psychiatric asylum, whether public or private, had to be reported to the criminal records office (*art. 604*). Such a link was to be weakened only in 1968 with the approval of the 'Mariotti law', which introduced voluntary admission to the psychiatric hospital and removed the obligation to notify the criminal records office on admission.

'Custodialism' and the dominant organicism created a strong therapeutic pessimism in the Italian asylum and in Italian psychiatry in general. Until the mid-1950s and the appearance of the first effective antipsychotic drugs, it was commonly accepted that 'di terapeutico c'è poco da fare' (Colucci and Di Vittorio, 2001: 19), an 'inanità terapeutica' (Girone, 1953: 157) that shocked many.

Basaglia came to know the asylum and its harsh reality only in 1961, when he moved to Gorizia. However, notwithstanding the milder conditions of the university clinic in Padua, Basaglia soon became dissatisfied with its uncritical attachment to a biological psychiatric model. Even in the gentler regime of the university clinic, the physician treated the patient as an object of study, whose psychiatric disease had to be observed, classified according to an established nosology and, if possible, treated accordingly. As Civita (1999: 90) remarks, 'l'interesse è rivolto esclusivamente alle proprietà del sintomo che possono essere accertate e descritte a prescindere dal contenuto strettamente individuale del delirio'. There was no interest (or at least a very limited interest) in the peculiarities of each individual patient, their histories, their lives and the context in which the mental illness arose. In other words, as Civita (1999: 93) puts it, there was no interest in the mentally ill person, only in mental illness as an object to be studied and treated in a medical context.

Alternative Psychiatries

There were few alternatives to such an organicistic and 'custodialistic' approach available in early-1950s Italy. Arguably, the main ones were psychoanalysis and so-called social psychiatry. Basaglia did not rely on either, at least not during his first years of practice in Belloni's clinic, for simple reasons. He was hostile to psychoanalysis: at first, Basaglia (1953a: 6) believed that psychoanalysis rests on a reductive organicist perspective, as it ultimately traces the whole psychic dimension back to primal instincts (Freud's *Trieb* – the drive), thus failing, like biological psychiatry, to understand mental illness beyond the organic nature of the human being. Later on, during his more politically engaged struggle to dismantle the asylum, he stressed how psychoanalysis is a classist science, devoted to the treatment of the minor ailments of the rich (bluntly, psychoanalysis is a very long and expensive treatment), thus it cannot possibly be of use in an institution such as the asylum (Basaglia, 1978b: 349–50 *passim*). Limited as this criticism may seem, it was enough for Basaglia not to engage with psychoanalytical approaches.

Conversely, social psychiatry, with all its variants, such as Maxwell Jones's 'therapeutic community', group psychotherapy, community rehabilitation centres, and so on, which were introduced in the United Kingdom during the final years of World War II, was almost unknown in Italy until Basaglia himself began, at a later stage in his career, to develop an interest in it.

To all intents and purposes, the only alternative available to Basaglia was a trend in psychiatry that had been around since the 1910s but which had few followers in Italy, at least until the psychiatrist Danilo Cargnello,

Basaglia himself, and other lesser-known psychiatrists such as Bruno Callieri and Eugenio Borgna, adopted it: phenomenological psychiatry, a trend that, in the 1950s, influenced not only Basaglia, but also Michel Foucault in his earliest writings as a psychologist, and the Scottish psychiatrist R.D. Laing, one of the main participants in the 1960s–1970s anti-psychiatry movement.[10] Phenomenological psychiatry, whose best-known founders were, among others, Karl Jaspers (1883–1969) and Ludwig Binswanger (1881–1966), is an 'umbrella' notion that unites different perspectives insofar as they all regard psychiatric symptoms as manifestations (phenomena) of the human being as a whole (not only of the biological/organic nature), whilst avoiding the systematisation of diseases into a nosology, their explanation, and the search for their essence and aetiology. In brief, phenomenological psychiatry posits that

> la malattia psichica non è un'entità separabile dalla storia di vita del paziente, [...] la malattia pertanto deve essere immersa e dispiegata nella trama e nel movimento complessivo della sua vita. (Civita, 1999: 93)

If the mandate of biological psychiatry was to study mental illness in its alleged organic causes, phenomenological psychiatry required understanding patients in their uniqueness. Possibly for this reason, the epistemological premises of phenomenological psychiatry were grounded much more in the philosophical tradition of Husserl's phenomenology and Heidegger's existential analysis than in the traditional medical approach of biological psychiatry.

---

10   For further historical and theoretical overviews of so-called phenomenological psychiatry see Galimberti, 2007 and Spiegelberg, 1972.

Towards Phenomenological Psychiatry

Jaspers' Phenomenological Psychopathology

One of the main epistemological differences between biological and phenomenological psychiatry amounts to the distinction between explanation and understanding, theorised by Wilhelm Dilthey (1833–1911) some decades before it was applied to psychiatry. In brief, Dilthey distinguishes between explaining [*Erklären*] natural facts and understanding [*Verstehen*] human subjects. He does this in order to valorise human beings beyond their factual and natural existence and in order to give 'human studies', such as psychology and history, the same methodological dignity as the 'physical sciences'. According to Dilthey (1976: 88), explanation, the methodological approach of the physical sciences, aims at 'subsum[ing] a range of phenomena under a causal nexus by means of a limited number of unambiguously defined elements'. Human studies

> differ from the [physical] sciences because the latter deal with facts which present themselves to consciousness as external and separate phenomena, while the former deal with the living connections of reality experienced in the mind. (Dilthey, 1976: 89)

Hence human sciences are 'based on mental connections' which, although we might as well be able to explain, we should also and especially *understand*:

> We explain nature but we understand mental life. Inner experience grasps the processes by which we accomplish something as well as the combination of individual functions of mental life into a whole. The experience of the whole context comes forth; only later do we distinguish its individual parts. This means that the methods of studying mental life, history and society differ greatly from those used to acquire knowledge of nature. Any empiricism which foregoes an explanation of what happens in the mind in terms of the understood connections of mental life is necessarily sterile. (Dilthey, 1976: 89)

Even if the physical nature of humans cannot be overlooked, a study of the human being cannot be limited to studying the physical nature of the organic body, for instance explaining mental states exclusively in terms of brain chemistry. A study of the human being must proceed from the understanding of mental processes rather than their explanation.

Karl Jaspers was the first to apply the Diltheyan distinction to psychiatry when, in 1913, he published the first edition of his very successful *Allgemeine Psychopathologie* (Jaspers, 1963). With *General Psychopathology*, Jaspers *de facto* founded the phenomenological trend in psychiatry, in that he required a discipline that 'non cerca le "cause" della follia nella genericità dell'organismo, ma il suo "senso" per il singolo individuo' (Galimberti, 2005: 302). From the outset, Jaspers (1963: 53) points to the centrality in psychopathology of phenomenology, understood as 'the study which describes patients' subjective experiences and everything else that exists or comes to be within the field of their awareness'. Hence, in studying mental illness, Jaspers attempts to overcome – at least partially – the pursuit for causal nexuses, the search for an organic aetiology or the classification of syndromes in an objective and super-individual way: in Husserl's wake, he seeks understanding of subjective phenomena as experienced by the patients themselves, the '*subjective* data of experience [which] are in contrast with other *objective* phenomena, obtained by methods of performance-testing, observation of the somatic state or assessment of what the patients' expressions, actions and various productions may mean' (Jaspers, 1963: 53). A psychopathological study, for Jaspers, cannot begin with the detached anamnesis sought by biological psychiatry; it must rather begin by establishing an immediate contact with the patient's subjectivity:

> Phenomenology sets out on a number of tasks: it *gives a concrete description* of the psychic states which patients actually experience and *presents* them *for observation* [...] Since we never can perceive the psychic experiences of others in any direct fashion, as with physical phenomena, we can only make some kind of representation of them. There has to be an act of empathy, of understanding [...]. Our chief help in all this comes from the patients' *self-descriptions*, which can be evoked and tested out in the course of personal conversation. [...] An experience is best described by the person who has undergone it. Detached psychiatric observation with its own formulation of what the patient is suffering is not any substitute for this. (Jaspers, 1963: 55; original emphases)

Thus, when the Diltheyan methodological distinction is applied to psychiatry, understanding and explanation become 'technical terms that represent two opposed approaches to a comprehension of human behaviour' (Phillips, 2004: 180). On the one hand, explanation aims at working out the functional and causal relationships between the data given by the patient: Jaspers calls this 'explanatory psychology', *Erklärende Psychologie*. The 'psychology of meaningful connections' (*Verstehende Psychologie*), on the other hand, points at 'sink[ing] into the psychic situation and understand[ing] genetically by empathy how one psychic event emerges from another' (Jaspers, 1963: 301). However, in spite of being a milestone in phenomenological psychiatry, for introducing the centrality of 'understanding' into psychiatry, Jaspers' *General Psychopathology* does not propose to abandon 'explanation' *tout court*:

> It is a mistake to suggest that the psyche is the field for the understanding while the physical world is the field for causal explanation. Every concrete event – whether of physical or psychical nature – is open to causal explanation. There is no limit to the discovery of causes and with every psychic event we always look for cause and effect. *But with understanding there are limits everywhere.* (Jaspers, 1963: 305; original emphasis)

Understanding, as a methodological approach in psychiatry, reaches its limits with psychoses such as schizophrenia: their symptoms are not understandable by the psychiatrist, who has to rely on causal analysis in such cases. As the Italian philosopher Galimberti (2007: 185) puts it,

> Jaspers non va oltre la determinazione del limite tra ciò che è 'comprensibile' e ciò che è 'incomprensibile' in un particolare uomo che si riveli alienato secondo i principi della psicologia esplicativa.

Jaspers indeed introduces the Diltheyan understanding in psychiatry, yet he also limits its possibilities. Hence, as Kimura (1982: 173–74) aptly notes:

> Phenomenology, as introduced by Jaspers, represents no more than a descriptive psychology in the sense of an empirical science. It remains far removed from the Husserlian phenomenological concepts such as the eidetic and transcendental reduction, or even the intuition.

In Jaspers' case, the limits of a phenomenological approach in psychiatry are clear: understanding of the subjective 'meaningful connections' – the data of phenomenology, according to him – is limited by psychotic states. In these cases understanding must subside and give way to an explanatory approach.

Binswanger's Daseinsanalyse

In his critique, Galimberti echoes Jung's student, Ludwig Binswanger (1881–1966), who sees the limits of Jaspers's psychopathology and tries to overcome them by creating a psychiatric research method known as *Daseinsanalyse* (or phenomenological anthropology). At the theoretical core of Binswanger's *Daseinsanalyse* lies Heidegger's *Sein und Zeit*, especially the first part, dedicated to existential analysis, which also kindled the philosophical current of existentialism.[11] To put it simply, the human being is, according to Heidegger, the only entity that inquires about its own being. The fundamental characteristic of this entity is to be always situated inside a world (the spatial surroundings, other people, external events, etc.), and in an inextricable and constant relationship with it. Heidegger calls 'this entity which each of us is himself' (Heidegger, 1967: 27) and who inquires about his own being *Dasein*,[12] literally there-being, *Da-Sein*, to stress the

---

11 Heidegger dedicated the first part of *Being and Time* to *Existenziale Analytik*, that is, to the analysis of the *Dasein*'s modalities of existence. This first part was not meant to be an independent method of studying humanity but a preliminary investigation into an ontology. Heidegger's main philosophical goal was to question Being as such, therefore *Existenziale Analytik* is not meant to be an anthropology. On the contrary, it is a study of man's ontological structure, which Heidegger calls *Dasein*; that is to say, man's relationship with his own Being and his own existence, as a privileged means to address Being as such. Both existentialism and *Daseinsanalyse* use Heidegger's existential analysis as an anthropology, leaving aside most of Heidegger's ontological reflection proper. See Heidegger, 1967: 67–77.

12 The word *Dasein* is a German expression, composed of the verb *sein* (to be) and the particle *da*, which has both a temporal (now) and a spatial (here) connotation. Heidegger uses *Dasein* in *Being and Time* to define man's ontological structure.

constitutional and constitutive relationship that it entertains, on the one hand, with being and, on the other, with the world, with his 'being-in-the-world' [*In-Der-Welt-Sein*].

The analysis of the *Dasein*, *Daseinsanalyse* in Binswanger's terms, requires psychiatry to approach every patient in his/her uniqueness, with a special attention to his/her 'situatedness': the biography, the modalities of one's relating to one's own world, etc. Hence, *Daseinsanalyse* begins from a radically different premise compared to Jaspers' psychopathology: both the 'sane' and the 'insane' can be understood, in that both – however differently – are in the world and are in a constitutional and constitutive relationship with their Being. Binswanger's *Daseinsanalyse* gives psychiatry:

> la possibilità di comprendere tanto l'′alienato' quanto la persona 'sana' come appartenenti allo stesso 'mondo', quantunque l'alienato vi appartenga con una struttura di modelli percettivi e comportamentali differenti. (Galimberti, 2007: 223–24)

In relying on Heidegger's existential analysis, Binswanger is able to distance himself from the pessimism of Jaspers' psychopathology, which ends up regarding psychotic behaviour as not being understandable. At the same time, Binswanger can also employ a phenomenological approach in psychiatry beyond Husserl's own somewhat limited application of phenomenology to psychology. As Galimberti (2007: 206) says:

> Husserl ha limitato la sua indagine al senso che si produce nel dispiegamento degli atti intenzionali, ma non ha detto nulla del modo d'essere della persona che compie questi atti.

Binswanger intends to formulate an analysis which is capable of accounting not only for the subject's acts but also, and above all, for the subject as such. An existential analysis of the *Dasein*, more than an approach exclusively grounded in Husserl's phenomenological psychology, can account for both the subject's acts and the subject's relationship with itself and the surrounding world.

Of all these considerations, what fascinates Basaglia the most is undoubtedly the new approach to the patient that stems from them.

Mainstream biological and institutional psychiatry, aiming at the explanation of symptoms rather than the understanding of the patient, encourages the formation of a detached relationship, as Jaspers called it, where the physician can treat the patient as an object of knowledge, to be studied as such. Biological psychiatry looks for a relationship between a subject (the psychiatrist) and an object (the patient). In opposition to this stance, Binswanger, who regards the gnoseological split between subject and object as the 'cancer of all psychologies and philosophies', proposes the idea of an 'encounter' between the psychiatrist and the patient, where both subjectivities could be called into question. Binswanger's encounter takes place between two subjects.

According to him (1962: 171), there are only two ways to practise psychiatry and to approach the patient:

> one leads away from ourselves towards theoretical determinations, i.e. to the perception, observation, and destruction of man in his actuality, with the aim in mind of scientifically *constructing* an adequate picture of him (an apparatus, 'reflex mechanism', functional whole, etc.). The other leads 'into ourself'. (original emphasis)

This second way, *Daseinsanalyse*, begins with the recollection of the patient's history. Through a discussion of the data collected, the psychiatrist opens up to the patient an understanding of one's self as a human being that should allow one to find one's 'way back' from the pathological state. Therefore, the psychiatric colloquium, rather than an anamnesis, is basically an encounter with a fellow human being.

At first glance such a stance could remind one of psychoanalysis: both *Daseinanalyse* and psychoanalysis begin with the recollection of the patient's history and favour open dialogue over a strictly medical process of anamnesis. Yet Binswanger, despite his friendship with Freud, dissociates himself from psychoanalysis.[13] According to Binswanger (1957b: 89), Freud's doctrine is of a 'monumental one-sidedness [in that it] interprets

---

13   As is testified to in their correspondence, collected in the volume Freud and Binswanger, 2000.

man only in terms of his natural characteristics'. Despite the fact that this assumption is at the very least arguable, Binswanger's *Daseinsanalyse* is conceived as a method for understanding human beings in their entirety, without limiting the analysis to what he called the 'homo natura' (Binswanger, 1957a). Basically, Binswanger's objection to Freud's psychoanalysis rests on its tendency to reduce human beings to their biological nature, analysing all human forms of expression, i.e. art, myth, religion, and so on, 'as reducible to their biological bases' (Bühler, 2004: 41); that is to say, in terms of drives. Yet drawing a clear-cut division between *Daseinsanalyse* and psychoanalysis is, to say the least, problematic. To a certain extent, it could be argued that both adopt very similar methods, i.e. the analysis of the patient's history, in order to achieve a rather similar goal, i.e. some kind of reconfiguration, rediscovery or reappropriation of the patient's subjectivity. The alleged psychoanalytic reduction of human beings to their nature is, to say the least, debatable and this problematises the very assumption of Binswanger's critique of psychoanalysis. The main difference between *Daseinsanalyse* and psychoanalysis could rest rather on the theoretical framework they adopt: one is grounded in Heidegger's existential analysis, the other in Freud's theory. Given that this is not the place to examine this complex relationship, suffice it to say that Basaglia's initial doubts about psychoanalysis are based on Binswanger's critiques. In Basaglia's words (1953a: 6),

> la scuola psicoanalitica portò in campo l'istinto e l'importanza di esso nel determinismo dei moti umani; tuttavia si partiva sempre dall'uomo come tale, o meglio dalla sua natura, facendo parte di essa pure l'istinto, attributo della natura umana, non sua manifestazione. [...] Si ricadeva quindi, anche se in una visione più ampia e più dinamica, in un concetto prettamente naturalista.

To conclude this section, it is important to specify that Binswanger did not necessarily mean *Daseinsanalyse* to be regarded primarily as a therapeutic method. As Spiegelberg (1972: 228) suggests, 'Binswanger saw limits to therapy and he looked upon the eventual suicide [of one of his clinical cases] as a kind of liberation and answer to an insoluble conflict': hardly a positive therapeutic outcome. *Daseinsanalyse* is not, primarily, a therapeutic method, but a means of studying and investigating mental phenomena as they manifest themselves in the human being regarded as a psychosomatic unity, always-already situated in a world: to some extent it does not matter whether this human being is mentally ill or not. For this reason, while Basaglia found a source of inspiration in Binswanger's work, he eventually parted company with *Daseinsanalyse*.

CHAPTER 2

The Subject and the Body

Introduction

Having contextualised Basaglia's work in Chapter 1, in this chapter I focus especially on those of his writings that show a clear influence of phenomenological psychiatry and existentialism, with the aim of presenting Basaglia's notion of subjectivity. From Basaglia's writings it can be understood that he envisions the subject, the individual and ultimately the person as intrinsically, always-already situated in a world and in a constitutional and constitutive relationship with all other people, with 'the other'.[1] In brief, Basaglia establishes a logical and ontological primacy of intersubjectivity over subjectivity: there is no subject outside of a world. The privileged pole around which this constitutional relationship is established is the body, which makes one aware of 'being oneself', and of the presence of the other, by projecting one into the world. Through the body one can

---

1   It is important to note that throughout the following sections I will use the terms 'individual' and 'subject' almost interchangeably, in accordance with Basaglia's use. I will leave an analysis of the distinction between individuality and subjectivity in Basaglia's often undistinguishable use of the terms to the final chapter of this book. Furthermore, Basaglia often resorts to terms such as *sé* (self) and *io* (I and ego). It is critical to note that, for the time being, these two terms are used neither with a Foucauldian connotation nor with a psychoanalytical one (i.e. the self is not regarded as the product of self-disciplining techniques and the ego is not considered as the product of an identification). 'Self' and 'I' are understood with a generic meaning: 'self' indicates the object of the reflexive relationship (one perceives oneself as 'self' in a reflexive relationship) and *io* (I or ego) is the subject of an action when this subject coincides with the subject of the utterance.

not only be aware of the world that surrounds one, but also of 'oneself' as a unique individual, setting oneself against the background of all other people. The aim of this chapter, therefore, is to unravel Basaglia's notion of a constitutional and constitutive tripartite relationship between the subject, the body and the other.

To being with, Basaglia's engagement with mainstream biological psychiatry, with phenomenological psychiatry and especially with *Daseinsanalyse* and Eugène Minkowski's approach must be discussed. These sections focus on the years 1953 and 1954 and develop two main topics: the embryonic outline of the logical and ontological primacy of intersubjectivity over subjectivity and the new relationship between psychiatrist and patient that Basaglia advocates.

The tripartite relationship between subject/body/other proper is then analysed, with particular focus on the years 1954–67. In these writings four main points emerge. While the subject is in a constitutional and constitutive relationship with the other and with the body, which Basaglia incarnates in the notion of the 'lived body', there has to be a *gap*, an *intervallo* between the subject and the other that somehow preserves the subject from promiscuity. The impossibility of establishing this gap might be a sign of or else engender a mental illness, but it might also be the effect, which Basaglia calls the 'institutionalised body', of the very psychiatric institution that was created to cure mental illnesses. As Pizza (2007) observes, the notion of the institutionalised body is a bridge between Basaglia's early interest in the subjectivity of the patient and his latter socio-politically engaged work of reforming psychiatry and ultimately closing the asylum. Through his reflection on the body Basaglia introduces into his psychiatric approach a number of socio-political considerations, integrating into his early *Daseinsanalytik* stance a number of notions that bring him remarkably close, as I endeavour to show, to Michel Foucault, among other thinkers.

The Young Basaglia and Phenomenological Psychiatry

'Il filosofo Basaglia'

When Basaglia turns for the first time to philosophy and phenomenological psychiatry it is not with the intention of rejecting institutionalism and biological psychiatry and replacing them with a new, more humane and humanistic approach to mental illness. The first contributions of 'il filosofo' Basaglia – as Belloni apparently nicknamed him for his interest in phenomenological psychiatry (Colucci and Di Vittorio, 2001: 2) – do not mark a break with the university or with biological/institutional psychiatry. Although scholars seldom mention it, Basaglia's early writings clearly show his initial agreement with mainstream biological psychiatry, especially with regard to clinical approaches, diagnosis and treatment. Important indicators of this agreement can be found in most of the articles from his phenomenological phase, up until the onset of his anti-institutional tendencies; that is, well beyond the first six papers, which were declaredly concerned with more traditional psychiatric matters such as barbituric subnarcosis (Basaglia and Rigotti, 1952), drawing tests (Basaglia, 1952) or verbal association tests (Basaglia, 1953b).

For instance, in the 1953 text 'Il mondo dell'incomprensibile schizofrenico' Basaglia (1953a: 12–13) presents the case of 'C. Rita, 25 years old, clinical diagnosis: schizoidia'[2] and analyses it by applying to the letter Binswanger's *Daseinanalyse*. Yet he comments that:

> la terapia biologica che certamente ha contribuito a riorganizzare il suo equilibrio organico è stata senz'altro utile a ridarle una certa stabilizzazione, a rafforzare il pur debole equilibrio psicologico creato dal suo ricovero, così da far nascere in lei la speranza di poter 'cominciare di nuovo', piena di un desiderio a lei sconosciuto di affrontare il mondo che fino allora aveva subito. (Basaglia, 1953a: 21)

2   Schizoidia is a term introduced by E. Bleuler (1857–1939) to indicate the tendency to turn towards the inner life, thus withdrawing from the external world (especially from society); see Campbell, 2009: 872.

The 'biological therapy' to which Basaglia (1953a: 13) refers is a series of twenty induced insulin comas.[3] Basaglia treats several other cases with shock therapies, as reported, for instance, in 'Contributo allo studio psicopatologico e clinico degli stati ossessivi' (Basaglia, 1954a: 86–89) and 'Il corpo nell'ipocondria e nella depersonalizzazione. La struttura psicopatologica dell'ipocondria' (Basaglia, 1956b).

This is an example of how Basaglia, in the first writings of his phenomenological phase, regards phenomenological psychiatry (here referred to as *antropofenomenologia*) as an ally of mainstream biological psychiatry (here referred to as *psicopatologia*) rather than as an opponent:

> psicopatologia e antropofenomenologia, se associate, si arricchiscono e si influenzano vicendevolmente: la psicopatologia in un senso di rapporto psicofisico, l'antropologia studiando come l'uomo si rapporti al suo prossimo attraverso la comunicazione, ricercando le relazioni di lui con il suo corpo e nello stesso tempo con se stesso. (Basaglia, 1957: 104)

As a matter of fact, although later in his career Basaglia would completely reject all forms of institutionalism in psychiatry – internment in the asylum, physical restraint of patients, uniforms to distinguish patients from doctors and nurses, etc. – he would never completely reject the assumptions of biological psychiatry. For instance, unlike most of the 1970s antipsychiatrists, Basaglia never denied that psychiatric suffering has to be regarded, to all effects and purposes, as an illness, an illness that might also have organic roots. On the one hand, his criticism is against all forms of biological reductionism: mental illness might well be an organic illness but it is *not only* an organic illness. On the other, he stands up against the institutionalism that is often implicit in biological psychiatry: the detached relationship between physician and patient, passing off as a 'cure' the use of shock therapies and sedative cocktails to render asylum inmates docile, and so forth. I will come back to this later. For the time being, suffice it

---

[3] The so-called insulin coma therapy is a shock therapy introduced by Manfred Sakel in 1933. It entailed overdosing the patient with insulin so as to induce a critical hypoglycaemic state and a controlled coma; see Campbell, 2009: 513–14.

to say that, initially, Basaglia resorts to phenomenological psychiatry to enrich the otherwise narrow and restrictive biological and institutional approach in psychiatry.

'Il mondo dell'incomprensibile schizofrenico'

Basaglia's 'declaration of committment' to a philosophical approach to psychiatry and, specifically, to *Daseinanalyse*, is formulated in the 1953 article 'Il mondo dell'incomprensibile schizofrenico' (Basaglia, 1953a), which is the first article in his *Scritti* (1981). Referring to Jaspers, Basaglia (1953a: 3) describes his method as follows:

> l'indagine fenomenologica si compie attraverso la percezione interna e non attraverso un processo di introspezione [...] L'analisi fenomenologica si ottiene [...] dalla descrizione, la più fedele possibile, delle esperienze soggettive del malato e dalla loro classificazione, una volta che l'esaminatore abbia presentato dette esperienze al suo spirito, immedesimandosi nella vita del malato stesso.

From the outset it is clear that, for Basaglia, the most important outcome of the application of phenomenology to psychiatry is a new clinical relationship: psychiatrists call into question their own world and choose to understand patients rather than explain their symptoms.

This new relationship is a 'relazione di comprensibilità' (Basaglia, 1953a: 4), where 'understandability' is read with a Diltheian interpretation. Following Jaspers, Basaglia regards 'understanding' as a direct subjective experience, as opposed to 'explanation' which requires a split between a subject who explains and an object for which an explanation is sought. We can understand, for instance, continues Basaglia, in Jaspers' wake, that a man who is insulted becomes angry and that a deceived lover becomes jealous (Basaglia, 1953a: 4). Yet this explains neither the mental state they are in nor how they got into that state. Explaining a psychic phenomenon 'non può cadere sotto il controllo soggettivo dell'esaminatore', whereas 'la comprensibilità ne è una diretta emanazione' (Basaglia, 1953a: 4).

Nonetheless, Jaspers's phenomenological psychopathology is, according to Basaglia, rather limited: it can approach psychic phenomena from an intersubjective perspective but it cannot grasp 'la totalità dell'essere umano' (Basaglia, 1953a: 5). The analysis of such totality, possible only in terms of Binswanger's *Daseinanalyse*, focuses on 'la vita particolare dell'uomo, tale quale esso è posto nel mondo' (Basaglia, 1953a: 5): its focus is not only the patients' subjectivity but also, and especially, the world they live in and their relationship with it.

This observation contains the key idea that there is no subject without and outside of a world. In the context of psychiatry, this conclusion has a fundamental consequence: psychiatric suffering is no longer read as the symptom of a dysfunction in the individual's organic nature but as a different, troubled or pain-provoking way of relating to the world. In agreement with Binswanger's stance, the analysis of the human being as a whole cannot proceed exclusively from their organic nature, an approach that Binswanger and Basaglia impute to biological psychiatry as well as to psychoanalysis. Focusing on biological nature, 'come principio di ogni cosa', ultimately surrenders psychiatric practice to a naturalistic and deterministic reduction of the 'manifestazioni infinite' of the human being to a 'legge preordinata [che] esist[e] in tutti i fenomeni naturali', the 'principî preordinati entro i quali la natura avrebbe posto l'uomo, la pianta, ecc.' (Basaglia, 1953a: 5*ff*). With a traditional biological approach therefore, psychiatrists cannot account for the variability of human beings and level their object of study, i.e. the patient, to *a priori* schematisms such as the traditional psychiatric nosology. Yet we cannot 'fissare nulla di determinato e di statico in ciò che è estremamente dinamico come la natura umana', says Basaglia (1953a: 7):

> Una pianta, una volta seminata, cresce e non potremo aspettarci mai delle grandi modifiche da ciò che è la legge generale; nell'uomo non succede così poiché egli nasce, cresce e muore, ma possiede un'altra fondamentale attività: l'intelletto con tutte le manifestazioni ad esso inerenti. Egli agirà e si esplicherà in manifestazioni infinite ed ognuna di esse sarà essenzialmente diversa da quella di un altro uomo, pur avendo con lo stesso un elemento fondamentale costituito dall'essere uomo [...] egli si esplicherà in svariate manifestazioni.

According to Basaglia, only an *a posteriori* 'phenomenological study' of the manifestations of human nature, focusing on the specificity of the singular subject, is capable of understanding the infinite possible paths that a human mind can follow in its experience. The psychiatric colloquium therefore, with its analysis of the patient's history, aims at reconstructing the specific way in which the patient exists (modality of existence) or at 'entrare nell'essere della persona ammalata e poter penetrare il suo modo di adattarsi alla nuova situazione determinata dalla malattia' (Basaglia, 1953a: 8).

In 'Il mondo dell'incomprensibile schizofrenico', Basaglia (1953a: 11) presents a clinical case, the twenty-five-year-old schizoid patient Rita, claiming that, thanks to *Daseinsanalyse*, it was possible to reach 'una comprensione del modo di essere [del soggetto] nella malattia'. Basaglia begins his analysis by looking at Rita's feelings of inferiority and distrust, which result in her inability to adapt to the world. Basaglia believes that Rita lacks confidence in her own *Dasein*; that is to say, she is unable to acknowledge and accept the constant dialectical relationship between being herself and being part of a world. Only when the subject accepts this dialectical relationship can she become an active participant in the world. Above all, this participation is crucial because, according to Basaglia, it is only in distinguishing herself from the rest of the world that the subject becomes an individual and gains self-awareness. Therefore, by withdrawing from the world, that is, by not accepting her being-in-the-world, Rita refuses the possibility of 'being herself'. In turn, unable to have any 'self-awareness', Rita cannot distinguish herself from the rest of the world. Rita does not know who she is; therefore she does not know where the world ends and where her self begins.[4] According to Basaglia, she is somehow 'falling' into the world and 'fading into it'. In Basaglia's own words (1953a: 14),

> quando l'esistenza non è sostenuta dalla possibilità di rapporto nel modo 'duale e plurale', essa non può rivelarsi al proprio *Dasein* come un 'esserci singolare' e non esistendo possibilità di rapporto dell'Io con se stesso (modo singolare) il soggetto è costretto a precipitare totalmente 'nel mondo'.

---

4   I am intentionally using a very generic vocabulary to describe Rita's condition, in line with Basaglia's paper.

Rita is unable to distinguish between the world and herself and this results in the two main symptoms of her schizoidia. The first is that her potentially unlimited existential possibilities shrink to what the world seems to dictate to her. She is unable to decide for herself, so she chooses according to what she believes the world wants from her. Secondly, she regards any change in the surroundings as a change in her own self. This condition is what Basaglia (1953a: 15) calls a 'rimpicciolimento della struttura esistenziale'.

Two points of consideration emerge from 'Il mondo dell'incomprensibile schizofrenico'. First, the analysis of Rita's case introduces the first reference to a new relationship between the psychiatrist and the patient, which I discuss in the next section. Secondly, the article itself anticipates Basaglia's notion of body, to which I return in the next half of his chapter. According to Basaglia, it is impossible to have an immediate relationship with one's self. Any form of self-knowledge and self-awareness must refer to an external world in order to be able to 'return' to the self. The impossibility of an immediate relationship between the individual and one's own self recurs often in Basaglia's early writings and is interwoven, as I show later, with Basaglia's notion of body. As we shall see, the body is the privileged pole through which individuals relate to themselves in such an indirect way. Further to this, as I argue in the following chapters, Basaglia implicitly retains throughout his work the idea that a human being is unable to 'become itself' – the ontogenesis of the self, which Basaglia (1956a: 167) calls the 'edificazione della persona' – outside of a relationship with the other, a characteristic feature of Basaglia's theory of the subject, which he shares with most existential philosophers and also with Foucault.

Despite the emergence of a new relationship with the patient, Basaglia never refers to a therapeutic process or to Rita's recovery, and this should be read in the context of the lack of therapeutic aims in Binswanger's *Daseinsanalyse*, to which I have already referred. The application of such a method can indeed produce a form of understanding of the patient's world but it does not guarantee or even facilitate any kind of recovery. In this article, Basaglia stresses the importance of considering mental illness as a different mode of existence rather than as an organic dysfunction that needs to be cured – although, it must be remembered, he praises the merits of insulin coma therapy and the advantages of treating Rita in the isolation of the asylum.

The Therapeutic Encounter

Basaglia develops his initial considerations of the new psychiatrist-patient relationship and the body, which conclude 'Il mondo dell'incomprensibile schizofrenico', in his next article, 'Su alcuni aspetti della moderna psicoterapia: analisi fenomenologica dell'incontro' (1954). Basaglia here deals with the concept of the 'encounter' on two different levels.

On one level, the encounter amounts to the constitutional dual structure of the *Dasein*, which is able to refer to itself only through the world, that is, through an external pole. Clearly, this understanding of the encounter derives from the impossibility of an immediate relationship with the self as expounded in 'Il mondo dell'incomprensibile schizofrenico'. Drawing on the Dutch phenomenological psychiatrist J.H. van den Berg (1914–2012), Basaglia considers the 'encounter' as a pre-reflexive unit, that precedes the 'Me' and the 'You' and thus creates the consciousness of a 'We' before the separation of the subjects. According to Basaglia (1954b: 35):

> soltanto nel momento in cui l'uomo sente la necessità di un rapporto umano egli diviene tale, in quel tanto che rompe il suo isolamento per entrare e darsi al mondo: [...] l'individuo che si isola perde la possibilità dell'incontro'.

Basically, the term 'encounter' stands here for the fact that human beings become such only in a relationship with others; that is to say, we find ourselves in a world and we are forced to entertain a relationship with it before becoming individuals and developing self-awareness.

Any possible alteration of the dual structure of the *Dasein*, the encounter, may result in a mental disorder, as is the case with Rita and the two studies Basaglia (1954b: 40–41 and 46–48) presents in 'Su alcuni aspetti della moderna psicoterapia'. Basaglia considers any alteration of the encounter, such as Rita's loss of self and her falling into the world, as a shrinking of the patient's existence, and thus of her possibilities of expression. This is the situation for both Rita and B.T., the priest whose case Basaglia discusses as the second study of 'Su alcuni aspetti della moderna psicoterapia'. B.T.'s existence 'shrinks' to a certain extent: he is unable to structure a relationship with the world (understood in the widest possible sense of the patient's surroundings, other people, events and even the physical space inhabited) and consequently is unable to set himself against the background of the world. He develops a mental disorder,[5] once again as a consequence of his 'debolezza nell'accettare l'ambiente come elemento determinante dell'"incontro"' (Basaglia, 1954b: 51).

The second interpretation of 'encounter' develops the new psychiatrist-patient relationship which Basaglia had already hinted at in 'Il mondo dell'incomprensibile schizofrenico'. In addition to representing one of the constitutional modalities of the existence of the *Dasein*, and also because of it, the notion of the encounter shapes the relationship psychiatrists should establish with their patients.

In the wake of Binswanger's idea of the encounter, Basaglia (1954b: 43–44) states that:

> il rapporto di autorità che potrebbe sussistere fra il personaggio del medico e quello del malato viene a sostituirsi con una relazione fra due strutture di individui che parlano assieme. [...] È [...] attraverso la ricostruzione del 'vissuto' dell'individuo esaminato che lo psicoterapeuta riuscirà a ridargli la possibilità di aprirsi e ritornare al mondo.

Language enables a privileged access to the encounter between the patient and the psychiatrist. Primarily, this means that psychiatrists should establish a basic linguistic understanding of the patients' world; that is, understanding their way of expressing themselves, their use of words, tone, register and gestures. Once psychiatrists have established this relationship, they can access the patients' world and their history. Psychotherapy can then begin on two different levels, for which Basaglia draws on Minkowski's (1970: 220–71) distinction between the notions of 'ideo-affective' and 'phenomeno-structural'. At first, therapy affects a patient's emotions, the

---

5   This mental disorder is defined by Basaglia (1954b: 46) as 'reazione fobico-ansiosa in psiconevrosi neuroastenica.'

affective level. The encounter is initially established on the basis of an understanding of the element that is shared between patient and psychiatrist, namely the fact of being human. The ideo-affective level of therapy amounts to an understanding of basic human feelings in their constitutional relationship with the individual. Interestingly, Basaglia argues that psychoanalysis also acts on this level. However, while psychoanalysis would ultimately dwell on this relationship (transference) as it intends to analyse it,[6] phenomenological psychiatry uses it as a basis for the encounter. Yet we should not expect this encounter to be a mere friendship:

> l'ammalato infatti non trova nel medico l'amico nel senso banale della parola, ma vede in lui la possibilità di risolvere se stesso attraverso un uomo che lo comprende (Basaglia, 1954b: 44).

Most importantly, therapy cannot be only ideo-affective, because this level is just one part of the human being's totality. Therapy must also act on a phenomeno-structural level. Psychiatrists need to make patients aware of their totality, which means making them aware that the pathological condition is an integrating part of their whole life. In other words, the final act of the therapeutic relationship is:

> [riportare] all'intera consapevolezza del paziente il meccanismo di formazione dei suoi disturbi, [ovvero rivivere] con il soggetto il modo nel quale si era posto nel mondo, lasciandolo libero di scegliere la maniera in cui egli doveva porsi durante e dopo il trattamento psicoterapeutico (Basaglia, 1954b: 52).

In spite of Basaglia's declared aversion for psychoanalysis, his approach is remarkably psychoanalytical. In brief, both Basaglia's approach and a psychoanalytical approach (understood in very generic terms without accounting for the different schools and currents in psychoanalysis) establish a relationship between the therapist and the patient on the grounds of a linguistic understanding, both focus on the study of patients' histories,

---

6   Basaglia has a rather limited grasp of the notion of 'transference', which he reduces to an 'identificazione da parte del soggetto della immagine detestabile paterna nella persone del psicoterapeuta' (Basaglia, 1954b: 44).

both (to a certain extent) bring patients to acknowledge the causes or at least the origins of their suffering and, finally, both leave patients 'free' during and after treatment, as Basaglia remarks in the above quotation. As Benvenuto (2005) points out, Basaglia's aversion to psychoanalysis is mostly ideological and often prevents him from adopting an established and unambiguously understandable vocabulary. In order to distinguish his own method from psychoanalysis, Basaglia often relies on vague descriptions of the psychiatric treatment, defending alternatives to psychoanalysis that sound remarkably similar to psychoanalysis itself but with an inconsistent use of terms such as 'I', 'subject', 'individual', 'world', 'other/s', and so on.

'Su alcuni aspetti della moderna psicoterapia' is once again an anticipation of concepts that Basaglia will only fully develop in his later work and the article is not without contradictions. As we have just seen, Basaglia does not adopt a consistent vocabulary in describing his practice and he always feels the need to differentiate his approach from biological psychiatry and psychoanalysis. Basaglia also shows a contradictory stance with regard to the idea of the patient and psychiatric practice. On the one hand, he is worried that 'il rapporto con il soggetto non sia da "psicoterapeuta a malato" ma da "psicoterapeuta a psicoterapizzato"' (Basaglia, 1954b: 43). On the other, he always refers to the patient as the sick person, 'il malato', to such an extent that he believes that 'l'Io dello psicoterapeuta deve sostituirsi all'Io del malato che non esiste più' (Basaglia, 1954b: 45), partially echoing the psychoanalytical school of ego psychology.

Apparently, the phenomenological encounter is still unable to deal with the relationships of power implicit in a mainstream biological and institutional psychiatric approach. Despite his desire to avoid any relationship of *authority* between the doctor and the patient, Basaglia does not question the persistence of relations of *power* inside his own method. Moreover, the concept of the encounter does not enable him to overcome the link between mental illness and error, abnormality and deviance. For instance, he refers to the pathogenetic moment as a 'sviata impostazione' (Basaglia, 1954b: 36) or, again, as a 'sbaglio iniziale' (Basaglia, 1954b: 51).

Nevertheless, the article features several important developments. First of all, Basaglia clearly advocates a new psychiatrist-patient relationship and he lays out its basic characteristics. We could consider it as his first expression of distrust towards the authority present in the biological/institutional psychiatric relationship.

Secondly, it becomes clear in this article that the Binswangerian 'way back' from mental illness, which consists basically of understanding patients' totality and sharing this understanding with them, is a strategy that must not stem from a predetermined psychiatric knowledge. That is to say, it is not through a rigidly rational and systematic nosological study of mental illness that we can approach the *incomprensibile* of psychosis. Reason cannot, in fact, account for its opposite and, therefore, an approach stemming from reason can only strengthen psychotic unintelligibility. Rather, the psychiatrist has to 'rintracciare la sua ragione [psicotica] e la chiave per accedervi' (Colucci and Di Vittorio, 2001: 30), a strategy that relies on the 'encounter' understood as a phenomenologically connoted notion. In these observations Basaglia refers for the first time, if only in passing, to the link between power and knowledge which will be crucial in his later works. This link will allow me to contrast and compare Basaglia with Michel Foucault in subsequent chapters. In fact, it is clear from these considerations that the authority implicit in the biological and institutional psychiatric relationship rests in and is justified on the grounds of a knowledge that remains external to the patient. The psychiatrist should seek knowledge *in* the patient's words rather than interpreting them on the grounds of previously constructed knowledge.

Finally, in 'Su alcuni aspetti della moderna psicoterapia', Basaglia gives his definition of the 'psychic':

> allorquando parliamo di 'psichico' non intendiamo riferirci necessariamente a qualche cosa di soggettivo ed individuale, poiché l'individuo partecipa oltre che di se stesso, di tutto ciò che lo circonda, [...] lo supera e investe tutte le altre entità umane, qualche cosa di interumano cui partecipa ogni essere. (1954b: 43)

The idea of the psychic dimension as something that surpasses the individual, a notion that is already evident in Basaglia's concept of the encounter as a constitutional structure of *Dasein*, further endorses the logical primacy of intersubjectivity over subjectivity and also plays an important role in the development of the concept of body, which I discuss in the following section.

The Subject, the Body and the Other

In previous sections, I have analysed Basaglia's preliminary considerations of the relationship between the psychiatrist and the patient and also his embryonic outline of a notion of subjectivity. In this section, I discuss Basaglia's later and more complex delineation of his theory of the subject. I argue that this theory develops the idea that there can be no direct relationship with the self. In brief, and also in the light of his phenomenological and existentialist influences, Basaglia advances the notion of a subject as always-already caught up in a constitutional and constitutive relationship with otherness. The ontogenesis of the self – the 'edificazione della persona' as Basaglia (1956a: 167) calls it; that is to say, the process of becoming a subject – entails the acceptance of being constantly (and paradoxically) at the mercy of the other, who has the power to intimately shape and determine us. Being an individual subject ultimately depends on acceptance of being caught up in this constitutive relationship with otherness. Outside of this 'relationality' there is no such thing as subjectivity and the possible outcomes of severing this connection – which would be attempted, paradoxically, to preserve individuality against the threat represented by the determining power of the other – can only result in psychosis.

Central to this notion of subjectivity is the concept of the lived body that Basaglia adopts from Merleau-Ponty. It is through the experience of the body that we become subjects in this paradoxical way: through the body we perceive ourselves as unique individuals but at the same time we are also forced to offer the body as an object to the other. Only by establishing such a vulnerable and ambiguous tri-polar relationship (the subject, the body, the others) is it possible to be (non-psychotic) subjects:

> Quando infatti l'individuo si corporeizza nel determinarsi come persona, quando cioè si contrappone al mondo esterno, deve possedere la rappresentazione di una unità, a volte psichica, a volte fisica, del proprio Io e, per far ciò, egli deve identificarsi e nello stesso tempo contrapporsi ai propri simili: è verso l'altro che egli dirige tutta la sua potenza affettiva ed è in questo altrui che egli si confonde e si immedesima (Basaglia, 1956a: 193).

The Lived Body

Giovanna Gallio remembers a gesture that Basaglia used to make when asked what the body was:

> lui univa il pollice con l'indice e tracciava un cerchio attorno al corpo, come un confine a una certa distanza, e diceva 'questo è il corpo'. [...] Il corpo, lui diceva toccandosi, non è qui, ma è nella traccia di questo cerchio che protegge il corpo come un'area di inviolabilità, ma anche come una linea di carcerazione. Questa traccia-confine non può riguardare un corpo solo ma, situandosi a metà, delimita il corpo dell'altro da cui prende senso. (quoted in Di Fusco and Kirchmayr, 1995: 82)

The body that this gesture evokes is very different from the body of medicine, the biomechanical and anatomical entity that can be opened up, dissected, divided into its interlinked components and explained in a functional and causal way. It is well established that the western philosophical tradition has tended to split the mere physical functions, the anatomical body, from the higher intellectual functions, the soul, conferring on the former an inferior and earthly value whereas the 'divine' and 'superior' character of the human being has been ascribed, along with consciousness, awareness, intellect and all psychic life, to the 'soul'. Such a dichotomy possibly originated with Plato's juxtaposition of the *soma/sema* (body/tomb) (see *Gorgias*, 493a; *Phaedrus*, 250c), feeding into Aristotle's notion of the body as an instrument for the soul (see *De anima*, II–1). Although the Aristotelian perspective bears less negative connotations than Plato's, it still puts the body (vegetative and animal functions) in an inferior instrumental relationship with the soul (the superior intellectual functions). Arguably, the most influential dichotomic model was advanced by Descartes with his split between *res cogitans* and *res extensa*. Within Cartesian dualism, body and soul and, later, body and mind, were firmly divided into separate entities, at least until Husserl's distinction between *Körper* (the body considered as an object of knowledge, the anatomical body) and *Leib* (the lived body, the body as it is perceived by the subject). With this distinction, the strict dualism body/soul (or body/psyche) is finally overcome: the lived body participates to all intents and purposes in the sphere of consciousness; that is to say, in the sphere of the psyche.

Basaglia's gesture in defining his idea of body somehow encloses this centuries-long debate: his gesture includes the actual physical body (Husserl's *Körper*), but it also describes an additional space around this physical presence, introducing Husserl's *Leib*. The body is not (only) mere flesh that can be opened up and exposed to the all-knowing (and all-discovering) gaze of the anatomo-pathologist – and in this, as I discuss in the fourth chapter, Basaglia seems to be anticipating Foucault's *The Birth of the Clinic* – but is also, and maybe especially as far as psychiatric practice is concerned, Husserl's *Leib*: the body as subjectively experienced, the threshold between subjectivity and otherness, between one's own self-perception, the other's perception of oneself and one's perception of the others. I will return to the notion of body as a threshold in the concluding chapter of this book, where I will focus on Esposito's notions of *communitas* and *immunitas* in relation to the body. For the time being, suffice it to note that the *Leib* is not an object for the pathologist's gaze: it plays the part of the protagonist in the sphere of subjectivity. It is not a body whose dysfunctions could generate mental illness. On the contrary, it is a body that can be distorted by mental illness.

I have already touched upon the fact that, throughout its history, psychiatry has sought a connection with the *Körper*: it sought it in brain lesions, the endocrine system, neuronal synapses, etc. Psychiatry has also always been interested in what is referred to as 'coenesthesis', which is the feeling of one's own body as it results from the merging of proprioceptive information and one's own spatial representation, in other words, the translation into conscious sensations of the vegetative functions of the organism (Basaglia, 1956b: 148). However, according to Basaglia, coenesthesis results in something more than the mere conscious rendering of the vegetative functions. Coenesthesis is the basis of the experience of one's own body, and it is during the translation process from organic sensations to lived experience that a pathological dysfunction can manifest itself.

The primacy accorded to the *Leib* rather than to the *Körper* and the importance of abandoning a 'concezione oggettivo-funzionale del corpo e considerarlo nel suo aspetto di vissuto' (Basaglia, 1956b: 162) marks the commencement of Basaglia's reflection on the 'lived body'. Openly echoing

The Subject and the Body

the phenomenologist Merleau-Ponty, Basaglia (1956b: 137) affirms that the body is not only

> oggetto complementare alla soggettività dell'Io, ma rappresenta [...] l'esperienza più profonda ed insieme la più ambigua delle percezioni: proprio questa ambigua bipolarità del corpo, contemporaneamente presente e dimenticato, soggetto ed oggetto delle percezioni, fa dell'esperienza corporea la più fragile delle esperienze.

According to Merleau-Ponty (2002: 230), 'the experience of our own body [...] reveals to us an ambiguous mode of existing'. Human beings cannot have an objective perception of their own bodies, hence 'my awareness of [my body] is not a thought' (Merleau-Ponty, 2002: 231). We have no other means of knowing a body, continues Merleau-Ponty (2002: 231), whether it is ours or another person's body, 'than that of living it'. In such a way, the very concept of body subverts the relationship between subject and object – and with it, the Cartesian body/mind split – in that the 'experience of one's own body runs counter to the reflective procedure which detaches subject and object from each other, and which gives us only the thought about the body [...] and not the experience of the body or the body in reality' (Merleau-Ponty, 2002: 231).

In drawing on Merleau-Ponty, Basaglia's theory of the subject is taking shape. According to him, there is no such thing as a subject that exists outside of the world, without being in a relationship with others. Likewise, it is not possible for any person to perceive their self as a self, distinct from the world, without setting that self against all other people. The body is the pole through which this constitutional and constitutive relationship between subjectivity and otherness becomes explicit: it makes one present to oneself by throwing one into the midst of other people.

On the one hand, the body enables one to relate to oneself. That is, the individual becomes aware of being an 'I', different and distinct from the rest of the world, only when one sets oneself as a body against the world.

Several mental disorders, such as depersonalisation and hypochondria contribute to the loss of this pole.[7] In the normal ontogenesis of the self it is

> nella contrapposizione fra Io e non Io [che] l'Io trova, nel legame con il corpo, la possibilità di opporsi al mondo esterno, giungendo in tal modo ad affermare se stesso. (Basaglia, 1956a: 171)

From this perspective, the lived body represents the privileged means of the subject's relationship with one's own self.

On the other hand, the lived body is also the privileged means of the relationship between the subject and the world. This is true insofar as the body is somehow that 'extension' of the subject which is given to the world. Or, in Basaglia's own words (1956a: 169), the lived body is a vehicle for being-in-the-world. Through the body, the sensations that come from the world reach consciousness. Consequently, when subjects do not relate to their body, or when this relationship is distorted, there can be no world or at least the world that results is misshapen. This is the case, for instance, in depersonalisation. In order to collect the sensations given by the world, the body has to make itself an object for the rest of the world. In becoming a subject, in setting itself against the world, in collecting the stimuli given by the world, the body 'aperto e vulnerabile, si staglia in mezzo agli altri e alle cose' (Basaglia, 1965a: 31).

---

7   Hypochondria is the obsessive belief that one has a severe illness, and is related to other minor manifestations such as an increased attention towards one's own bodily sensations. On the other hand, depersonalisation is a feeling of distance from one's own body, and eventually from the rest of the world. The subject perceives his body as not belonging to himself and feels excluded from the world. During the first years of Basaglia's practice, mainstream psychiatry did not categorise hypochondria and depersonalisation as mental illnesses. Rather, it considered both of them as symptoms of more complex neurotic or psychotic states. Psychiatrists often regarded hypochondria and depersonalisation as signs of an incipient psychosis (pre-psychotic manifestations).

'Alterità' and 'Alienità'

The subject can be in the world only if his/her body is always-already 'thrown' into it, understood in terms of Heidegger's *Geworfenheit*, 'thrownness', a central characteristic of the *Dasein*. According to Heidegger, the *Dasein* is always-already in a world, in a situation, cast into it since its birth, so much so that we cannot understand *Dasein* as an entity that precedes Being-in-the-world: the *Dasein* is, strictly speaking, the 'there' [*Da*] in which Being [*sein*] is always-already thrown:

> we call it the 'thrownness' of this entity into its 'there'; indeed, it is thrown in such a way that, as Being-in-the-world, it is the 'there'. The expression 'thrownness' is meant to suggest the *facticity of its being delivered over*. (Heidegger, 1967: 174)

'Thrown' into the world as a body, the subject, according to Basaglia, is in a constitutional and constitutive relationship with otherness: 'esistere significa essere per porsi con gli altri' (Basaglia, 1963: 8). It is when faced with the unavoidability of this relationship that the subject can choose an authentic existence or to fall into an inauthentic one. Following Heidegger's (1967: 312–48) thought, Basaglia bases his distinction between an authentic and an inauthentic *Dasein* on choice: an 'authentic existence' is, loosely put, when subjects choose and accept their existence fully and by themselves whilst maintaining a constant negotiation with others and with the world. Conversely, inauthenticity is the condition of the *Dasein* who falls into the impersonal 'They', delegating the choices of existence to others. In the impersonal 'They', 'everybody is the other, and no one is himself' (Heidegger, 1967: 165); that is to say, in the impersonal 'They' everybody is free to do only what everybody does. The impersonal 'They' homogenises the possibilities of one's existence and takes away responsibility of choice from the individual.

As Basaglia (1963: 6) remarks in 'Ansia e malafede', 'l'inautenticità è la mia incapacità a realizzare tutte le mie possibilità individuali in seguito alla mancata presa di coscienza di me'. However, becoming 'aware of oneself' does not entail a meditative act that would exclude others and make the subject perceive itself in some kind of solipsism, because

> l'uomo non può attuare [un] atto di riflessione su di sé se non attraverso lo sguardo altrui: è lo sguardo d'altri come intermediario che mi rimanda da me a me stesso che mi rende cosciente di me. (Basaglia, 1965a: 32)

Becoming 'aware of oneself' means to face the unavoidability of a relationship with others.

In the 1965 article 'Corpo, sguardo e silenzio', Basaglia (1965a: 31–33) posits that the relationship between the subject and the other can be either *alterità* (otherness) or *alienità* (alienity). The subject can choose to accept the presence of the other and with it the fact that were it not for this presence and its objectifying gaze the subject would not be able to be a subject at all (choosing *alterità*).[8] Otherwise, one could attempt to remove oneself completely from being exposed to the determining presence of the other. In this case, one would unfailingly fall into an (inauthentic) state of *alienità*. Here Basaglia echoes one of his primary sources of inspiration, Sartre's *L'être et le néant* (*Being and Nothingness*):

---

8   *Oggettificazione* and *oggettificare* are terms that Basaglia uses frequently. Lovell and Scheper-Hughes note that these terms might sound unorthodox in English and, in the introduction to the only collection of works by Basaglia translated in English, say: '*Objectify* is a term that Basaglia uses repeatedly. He is referring to the reification of patients and their afflictions through biomedical diagnosis and treatment. For Basaglia diseases (any more than patients) cannot simply be reduced to biological entities. Patients and illness speak to the sensitive and often contradictory aspects of culture and social relations. The objectivity of medicine and psychiatry is always a phantom objectivity, a mask that conceals more than it reveals' (Lovell and Scheper-Hughes, 1987: 7n). However, more generally, I would note that Basaglia also uses 'to objectify' and 'objectification' with reference to the normal and 'authentic' intersubjective relationship: thrown into the world the gaze of the other can objectify me as much as I can, the other way around, objectify the other: 'un soggetto oggettivizza l'altro nel momento in cui viene lui stesso oggettivato' (Basaglia, 1967a: 101). The problem with a traditional doctor-patient relationship is that objectification is not reciprocal. An authentic relationship, an 'incontro reale' between the psychiatrist and the patient should in fact 'presupporre una reciprocità in cui il terapeuta si troverebbe messo in discussione dal malato così come il malato è messo in discussione dal terapeuta' (Basaglia, 1967a: 101).

> I thereby recognize and affirm not only the Other but the existence of my Self-for-others. Indeed this is because I can not not-be the Other unless I assume my being-as-object for the Other. The disappearance of the alienated Me would involve the disappearance of the Other through the collapse of Myself. [...] But as I choose myself as a tearing away from the Other, I assume and recognize as mine this alienated Me. (Sartre, 1978: 285)

One cannot distinguish oneself from the other without assuming and accepting that one is at the mercy of the other, an object for the other. Removing oneself from the objectifying power of the other would entail the collapse of one's self.

Choosing *alterità* rather than *alienità* means to accept that one is at the mercy of the other but it also means, at the same time, establishing a *gap*, an *intervallo* between oneself and the other. Failing to maintain such a gap means one falls into a state of *alienità*, whereby the distinction between the subject and the world becomes blurred and the subject alienates itself in the other (Basaglia, 1965a: 31). The seemingly paradoxical feature of falling into a state of *alienità* is that the gap between the subject and the other collapses precisely when the subject attempts to make it insurmountable. In defending oneself to the utmost from the determining presence of the other, that is, by rejecting the constitutional relationship with others, there is no advent of subjectivity. There is, strictly speaking, no subject, no individual, no person: this is what Basaglia calls *alienità*, a state in which the non-subject is assaulted by others, in a condition of 'promiscuità in cui l'altro [...] urge senza tregua' (Basaglia, 1965a: 31).

The *gap*, the *intervallo*, that distinguishes *alterità* from *alienità* enables one to entertain a relationship with others without completely 'falling' or 'fading' into them. In the state of *alienità* there is no gap: one tries to distance the other completely, to be without others, and one is bound to fail.

> Nel momento in cui l'uomo perde l'occasione di vedersi, di accettarsi [...] attraverso l'oggettivazione datagli dalla presenza dell'altro, perde la possibilità di uscire dalla molteplicità per porsi in opposizione; perde dunque la reciprocità dell'incontro con l'altro che invade il suo spazio [...] l'uomo perde la propria alterità e si aliena. (Basaglia, 1965a: 37)

Establishing the gap that enables one to embrace the constitutional and constitutive relationship with otherness while at the same time not completely fading into the other necessitates the acceptance of the body as that physical 'extension' of subjectivity, that ambiguous and fragile experience which is always-already thrown into the world, at the mercy of the other's gaze:

> Se il mio corpo è la mia fattità, devo dunque accettare questa fattità, devo scegliermi come corpo per uscire dalla molteplicità e farmi uno. (Basaglia, 1965a: 31)

Here, Basaglia parts company with his first thoughts on the encounter. Following Binswanger, Basaglia first sought for a relationship able to uncover the *Dasein*'s original dual structure, the 'We' which precedes the idea of a divided 'I and You'. When it comes to defining the subject in terms of a constitutive relationship with others, Basaglia completely subverts this idea. As he remarks:

> è nel pormi chiaro e distinto di fronte ad un altro individuo che io mi scelgo in una lotta mia, in una mia scelta verso un fine, un futuro che è 'mio e tuo' prima che 'nostro'. (Basaglia, 1963: 7)

In departing from Binswanger's stance, Basaglia is here embracing Sartre's. Choosing *alterità* means several different and simultaneous things: it means accepting that one is constantly exposed to the other, establishing and negotiating a gap that allows the subject not to alienate into the other, and choosing one's own body as a fragile threshold. It means, in the general economy of the 'edificazione della persona', to become oneself whilst accepting that such a 'self' is always-already in a relationship with others. As Sartre posits, in a passage that was dear to Basaglia (it is the epigraph of 'Ansia e malafede'):

> The law of my freedom which makes me unable to be without choosing myself applies here too: I do not choose to be for the Other what I am but I can try to be for myself what I am for the Other, by choosing myself such as I appear to the Other. (Sartre, 1978: 529)

The whole edifice of the ontogenesis of the self depends on 'choosing oneself' as *alterità* or fading into the other in a state of *alienità*. As I discuss in the next section, the very definition of a mental disorder rests, according to Basaglia, on this distinction.

Psychosis and Neurosis

Falling into a state of *alienità* is for Basaglia a sign of mental suffering. In order to better understand the pathogenetic implications of the state of *alienità*, it is vital to refer to Basaglia's 1966 article 'L'ideologia del corpo come espressività nevrotica', where he dwells on the distinction between neurosis and psychosis,[9] openly drawing on the psychiatrist Heinz Häfner (1961).[10] According to Basaglia (1966a: 73), the neurotic subject suffers from a

9   Drawing a precise line of distinction between neuroses and psychoses would be impossible in the limited space available. Suffice it to say that, according to most of Freud's early works, neurosis is a mental ailment that pervades the internal psychic functioning of the subject: for instance, it could have originated in a repressed memory or desire. Psychoanalytic treatment is effective in dealing with neurosis in that it addresses the nucleus which contains the cause of neurosis: the unconscious. On the other hand, a psychosis pervades the subject's relationship with the outside world, his very perception of reality. As such it is almost inaccessible to psychoanalytical treatment. For instance, in his 'Neurosis and Psychosis', Freud (1924) clearly suggests that neurosis is generated by a conflict between the ego and the id, while psychosis is triggered by a conflict between the ego and reality. While Freud gradually abandons this position, and his successors, such as Karl Abraham (1927), adopt a more nuanced distinction between neurosis and psychosis, this dichotomy remains controversial even today, especially with the discovery of borderline states which define the state of an apparently neurotic subject who, during a treatment such as psychoanalysis, develops distinctly psychotic symptoms (Kernberg, 1975). For a study of the distinction between neurosis and psychosis see, for instance, Jacobson, 1972.
10 Heinz Häfner (born 1926) is a German psychiatrist, and director of the Central Institute for Mental Health in Mannheim. Häfner is responsible for the reform of psychiatry in Germany, which humanised psychiatric assistance and introduced a community-centred mental health care.

diminuita capacità [...] di fronteggiare le proprie istanze emotive, che lo urgono in modo tale da fargli perdere la spontaneità della propria esperienza corporea.

Unable as he is to 'vivere il proprio corpo immediatamente [...] nella fusione somatopsichica', and being the body the pole on which the intersubjective relationship is established, the neurotic tries to maintain a relationship with the other outside of an authentic condition of *alterità* by trying to build 'un'immagine [...] capace di legarlo [...] all'altro da cui non sopporta di essere escluso'. This is what Basaglia refers to, using Häfner's words, as 'espressività nevrotica' (Basaglia, 1966a: 73). Remaining 'nei limiti dell'ordinamento mondano', the neurotic tries to 'dominare le istanze che erompono, elaborandole come compromesso' (Basaglia, 1966a: 74). While the neurotic's 'azioni espressive' try to convey such 'erupting demand', this is bound to remain 'insoddisfatta, anche nel momento stesso in cui viene comunicata' (Basaglia, 1966a: 74). In passing, I would note that Basaglia seems here to be almost intentionally avoiding a comparison with psychoanalysis. The 'domande che erompono', 'erupting demands', arguably retain all the characteristics of unconscious desires according to Freud's formulation: the neurotic represses an unconscious desire which then returns expressed in the compromise formation of the symptom, because repression is never completely successful. The symptom is always a mere compromise and is therefore bound to be unsatisfactory insofar as it deviates from the original unconscious content that was to be expressed (Freud, 1923: 242).

On the other hand, psychosis is not expressive, that is, a psychotic symptom does not express an 'underlying erupting demand'. Psychotic actions are not 'azioni di espressività' but 'azioni di rottura psicopatica' (Basaglia, 1966a: 73): the distance from others 'deve essere mantenuta e l'azione di rottura è appunto espressione dello sforzo attuato per mantenerla' (Basaglia, 1966a: 74). By radically breaking with the other, psychotic subjects do not experience the distance between themselves and others as a space in which to realise themselves as subjects (the *intervallo* that allows human beings to be in an intersubjective relationship without losing themselves into the other). On the contrary, psychotic subjects completely lose their distance and precipitate themselves into the other: this is the apparently paradoxical outcome of Basaglia's theory of *alterità/alienità*. It is only by maintaining a *distance* from the other that one can acknowledge onself as, in turn, *other*. This *intervallo*, the gap between one and all other people enables one to establish the unavoidable relationship with the other: this is a state of *alterità*. Yet this distance cannot be a complete fracture with otherness because that would cause a state of *alienità*: by refusing to be in a relationship with the other (which, paradoxically, one would refuse precisely in order to safeguard to the utmost one's *distance* from the other, to make it insurmountable, to protect oneself from the other) one loses the *intervallo* and fades into the other. This was already clear in the 1953 article 'Il mondo dell'incomprensibile schizofrenico', where Basaglia (1953a: 15) defined this situation as the 'shrinking' of the psychotic existence. According to Basaglia (1965a: 36), the psychotic is 'devastato dallo sguardo dell'altro, dal mondo dell'altro che lo reifica, lo condensa, lo annulla', which is the psychotic outcome of what Basaglia, in Sartre's wake, calls a 'comportamento di malafede':

> Costantemente preoccupato di mantenere la distanza dall'altro che, altrimenti, entrerebbe in lui, presume di poterlo in questo modo determinare senza accorgersi che, proprio in questa costante, ossessiva necessità di distanziarsi egli è dall'altro dominato e determinato: si oggettivizza proprio quando crede di più soggettivarsi. (Basaglia, 1963: 10)

Both the psychotic and the neurotic have trouble with their *alterità* and therefore they fall into a state of *alienità*. While neurotic subjects alienate into an image, in the 'azioni di espressività nevrotica', which allows them to entertain an (inauthentic) relationship with the other, psychotic subjects completely break with otherness and, in refusing to be a part of it, are 'swallowed' by it.

The Institution and the Body

Mental illness is certainly not the only condition in which we can witness a state of *alienità* and with it a distortion, for lack of a better word, of the experience of the body, the lived body. Soon after dedicating his attention to the lived body, Basaglia was appointed director of Gorizia asylum (1961) and discovered that institutionalism and prolonged internment also, and maybe especially, affect the inmates so deeply, that they ultimately shape the inmates' very bodies. This is what Basaglia refers to as the 'institutionalised body'. In this notion he conflates his phenomeno-existentialist analysis of the lived body with a number of studies, the first and central of which is Barton's 1959 *Institutional Neurosis*. These studies demonstrate the negative effects that prolonged institutionalisation has on mental patients, debunking the centuries-old claim that isolation in the asylum is therapeutic in itself (William Battie originated this trend in 1758). In the notion of the 'institutionalised body' Basaglia is confronting an idea that is also central to Michel Foucault's work, although Foucault will fully develop it in writing only in his 1975 *Surveiller et Punir* (*Discipline and Punish*). I am referring here to the relationship between political power and the individual body. In *Discipline and Punish*, Foucault (1991: 138) notes how disciplinary power, which could be roughly defined as the direct exercise of power over individual bodies, actively 'produces subjected and practised bodies, "docile" bodies'. In the 1973–74 course at the *Collège de France*, *Psychiatric Power*, Foucault (2006b: 56), affirms that disciplinary power 'fits somatic singularity together with political power. What we call the individual is not what political power latches on to; what we should call the individual is the effect produced on the somatic singularity, the result of this pinning, by techniques of political power'. With his notion of the 'institutionalised body', Basaglia is referring precisely to such a connection between political power, the bodies of the inmates and their subjectivity.

This connection becomes clear for the first time in his 1966 paper 'L'ideologia del corpo come espressività nevrotica'. Here, he affirms that,

> il problema che si pone si concreta, in definitiva, in una sola domanda: se cioè l'alterata esperienza corporea del neurastenico non sia evidenza del suo vivere *ideologicamente* il proprio corpo e *quali legami possa avere una simile esperienza ideologica con la nostra realtà sociale* [added emphases]. (Basaglia, 1966a: 69)[11]

---

11 Basaglia here employs the term 'ideology' in a Marxist interpretation of 'false knowledge', referring especially to Karl Mannheim's definition. Ideology in such an interpretation is the primary means of alienation: the individual conceals from himself

In the 'normal' process of 'edificazione della persona', the individual chooses and lives his or her body as thrown into the world, exposed to the other's gaze, in order to be in a relationship with the world. In such an exposed condition, the body itself is shaped and reshaped: other people, social conventions, advertisements and public images, even *laws* shape our own experience of the body. This is why in a condition of *alterità* there needs to be an *intervallo*, small and feeble as it may be, that prevents us from completely alienating into the other.

This gap cannot be established in the psychiatric hospital. Once interned in an asylum, patients begin their 'moral career' as inmates. In the wake of the sociologist Erving Goffman (2007: 154), Basaglia stresses that once admitted to a 'total institution' such as an asylum, a prison or a hospital, the patient/inmate/prisoner is required to abandon their self and to identify completely with the institution. This begins with the inmate being exposed to the physical promiscuity of the asylum wards. Goffman (2007: 35) calls this promiscuity 'contaminative contact' because it is characterised by several, and often violent, impositions on the body: the obligation to take medicines, eat (or be force-fed) and especially to be completely controlled by others. In Goffman's words (2007: 35), the inmate 'is being contaminated by a forced relationship to these people [nurses, psychiatrists, other inmates, etc.]'. The inmate is thus regarded as nothing other than a *Körper* in Husserl's terms, a naked, anatomical body, a

> punto di passaggio: un corpo indifeso, spostato come un oggetto di reparto in reparto, cui viene impedita – concretamente ed esplicitamente – la possibilità di ricostruirsi un corpo proprio che riesca a dialettizzare il mondo, attraverso l'imposizione del corpo unico, aproblematico, senza contraddizioni dell'istituto. (Basaglia, 1967a: 110)

In medicine in general, Basaglia (1967a: 101) argues that 'l'incontro fra medico e paziente si attua nel corpo stesso del malato'. However, the body invoked as the third pole of the relationship between physician and

---

his poor conditions of life, idealising them. He appeals to absolute moral principles to justify his conditions, to the point that he does not want to fight and overcome them. See Mannheim et al., 1936.

patient is far from being conceived in terms of a 'lived body'. In Basaglia's words (1967a: 101), 'che il corpo visitato dal medico appartenga al soggetto specifico che lo vive e lo significa, ciò esula dalla finalità del rapporto che viene a instaurarsi'. The medical relationship is based on a 'corpo che si presume in qualche modo malato, operando un'azione oggettivante di carattere pre-riflessivo, da cui si deduce la natura dell'approccio da stabilire', and the consequence of such an approach is that it imposes on the patient/inmate 'un ruolo oggettivo sul quale l'intera istituzione che lo tutela viene a fondarsi', a role that 'finisce per influire sul concetto di sé del malato il quale [...] non può non viversi che come corpo malato' (Basaglia, 1967a: 102).

Psychiatry and its institutions originally sought to cure diseases yet, eventually, pave the way to the artificial fabrication of an image of the 'sick'. According to Basaglia, this image has no therapeutic or scientific value, and it only answers the need to justify and guarantee psychiatric knowledge by confirming it as an authoritative medical science: psychiatry 'nel suo costituirsi come metafisica dogmatica ha dovuto imporre e costruire nel corpo del malato la conferma delle proprie ipotesi' (Basaglia, 1967a: 100).

Forced into this 'objectified' and 'reified' condition, usually for many years, the asylum inmates eventually introject the image that the institution imposes on them and fully identify with a body in which the institution has entered (Basaglia, 1967a: 105–8). Basaglia describes the effects of the institutionalised body with an oriental tale: a snake enters the body of a man and deprives him of his freedom of choice. When eventually the snake leaves, the man is unable to live and act normally: he is no longer used to freedom and, consequently, does not know what to do with it.[12] According to Basaglia (1967a: 106), this tale is analogous with the institutional condition, in that

> il malato, che già soffre di una perdita di libertà quale può essere interpretata la malattia, si trova costretto ad aderire ad un nuovo corpo che è quello dell'istituzione [...]. Egli diventa un corpo vissuto nell'istituzione, per l'istituzione, tanto da essere considerato come parte integrante delle sue stesse strutture fisiche.

---

12   In Basaglia, 1967a: 105–6, Basaglia claims he first read the tale in *Il lavoro e la libertà* (Davydov, 1966).

Deinstitutionalisation, as I will show in subsequent chapters, must therefore begin by removing the 'snake' from the institutionalised psychiatric patient but cannot stop at this. Such an internal reform is the beginning of a number of initiatives that can only bring the reforming psychiatrist to the conclusion that the psychiatric hospital system has to be completely dismantled.

CHAPTER 3

The 1960s: Challenging Psychiatry

Introduction

In 1958, whilst working in Belloni's clinic, Basaglia became a lecturer at the University of Padua. Three years later, he left for the asylum at Gorizia but the reason why he did so is still a matter of debate. Possibly, Basaglia did not want to fall into the 'sindrome universitaria, quasi che l'intera esistenza si risolvesse soltanto in questa realtà: la carriera universitaria' (Basaglia et al., 1978: 103). Yet Basaglia himself gave this explanation only *a posteriori*, almost twenty years after leaving Belloni's clinic for the asylum. Giovanni Jervis, who worked with Basaglia and later strongly criticised his ideals, argues that Belloni fell out with the university and thus denied Basaglia the prospect of an academic career. According to this interpretation, Basaglia had to move to Gorizia where he lived 'malvolentieri, un po' come in esilio' (Corbellini and Jervis, 2008: 83). Another explanation comes from Basaglia's biographer, Michele Zanetti, a member of the provincial council that supported Basaglia's reforms in Trieste. Zanetti suggests that Belloni was on the verge of retiring and could not back Basaglia's academic career; hence, following the advice of his wife, Franca Ongaro, Basaglia accepted the post of director of Gorizia's asylum. Whatever the biographical reasons, Basaglia never completely endorsed Belloni's organicism. Possibly he was eager to find a less conservative *milieu* in which he could develop his own thoughts. Only at a later stage did he subject the university to a harsh critique.[1]

---

1 See, for instance, *Struttura sociale, salute e malattia mentale* in *Conferenze brasiliane*: 'l'università e la scuola [...] non insegnano nulla [...] sono solo un punto di partenza [...] prima di entrare nel gioco della produttività' (Basaglia, 2000: 91).

What matters most for the purpose of this research is that Basaglia's dissatisfaction with organicism turned, in Gorizia, into the shock of entering a total institution and encountering the institutionalised bodies of the inmates. Because of this shock, three years later, in 1964, at a conference in London, Basaglia made one of his best-known statements: 'la distruzione del manicomio è un fatto urgentemente necessario, se non semplicemente ovvio' (Basaglia, 1964a: 19), officially inaugurating his work of deinstitutionalisation.

However, it must be borne in mind that the 1960s were as much a period of great tumult in psychiatry as in society in general, and Basaglia's work, revolutionary as it was, cannot be considered outside of this context. Without being exhaustive, this chapter is devoted to outlining the main ideas of those who have often been improperly grouped under the label 'anti-psychiatrists', ideas which underpinned two decades (1960s–1970s) of worldwide protest against mainstream biological and institutional psychiatry. The first step to understand this movement in its social and historical context is to unravel the reasons why psychiatry came to be radically challenged in the 1960s. Having done so, the protagonists of this challenge and their ideas will be presented. The second half of the chapter is dedicated to one of these protagonists in particular, arguably the most influential: Michel Foucault. The analysis begins with *Histoire de la folie à l'âge classique*, his 1961 work on the history of madness, concluding with his groundbreaking formulation of disciplinary power as applied to psychiatry.

Psychiatry at the Beginning of the 1960s

Jervis observes that, in the late 1950s, mainstream biological and institutional psychiatry was experiencing a crisis. Psychiatry

> avvertiva il suo ritardo scientifico rispetto ad altre branche della medicina e soffriva della mancanza persistente di terapie efficaci contro i disturbi del comportamento. (Corbellini and Jervis, 2008: 36)

Yet the crisis was not so much caused by any scientific backwardness as by a number of socio-historical reasons. In the first place, the aftermath of the Second World War was casting a sombre light on psychiatry. A terrible truth about the Nazi 'Final Solution' had surfaced: many doctors, and psychiatrists especially, had collaborated in the *Shoah* and other forms of genocidal violence, and 'i malati di mente erano stati tra i principali obiettivi di discriminazioni sistematiche basate su pregiudizi biologistici, e ne erano nati abusi agghiaccianti' (Corbellini and Jervis, 2008: 41).

Psychiatry was also seen to have supported colonisation in many cases, and the abuses related to it. The psychiatrist Frantz Fanon, who studied the psychological effects of colonisation and racism in Algeria, pointed out that, 'the Algerian was a born criminal. A theory was elaborated and scientific proofs were found to support it' (Fanon, 1961: 239). This theory was grounded on dubious psychiatric studies such as that produced by the World Health Organization representative, Dr. A. Carothers, who believed that 'the African makes very little use of his frontal lobes' (Carothers, 1954: 176). According to Carothers, Fanon (1961: 244) continued, 'the likeness existing between the normal African native and the lobotomized European is striking'. Several other studies emerged, especially after 1954, linking psychiatry with colonialist regimes. A similar debate concerned the difficulties that arise 'when seeking to "cure" a native properly, that is to say, when seeking to make him thoroughly a part of a social background' (Fanon, 1961: 200). Psychiatry was therefore seen as a means by which to impose and enforce a social order, disguising the subjection and adherence to the regime as a medical cure. This holds good also for the political abuse in psychiatric hospitals (*'psikhushkas'*) perpetrated by the Soviet Union, in order to intern, silence and discredit political dissidents. However, this reality surfaced later, in 1971, when the Soviet human rights activist Vladimir Bukovsky smuggled papers to *The Times* documenting the use of psychiatry for political repression.[2]

---

2   See, for instance: Gersham, 1984; Bonnie, 2002; and also the review of Bukovsky's documents by the University of Sheffield (Richter, 1971).

Fanon uncovered the social role of psychiatry in a colony such as Algeria, and Bukovsky's documents concerned the Soviet Union. Jervis, among others, highlighted the link between Nazism and psychiatry. However, other scholars and psychiatrists in the 1960s focused on psychiatry as it was practised in Europe and in the United States, at the heart of western world. Notably, the role of psychiatry appeared to be rather similar to the one it played in colonialism or Nazi Germany, if milder, giving rise to a movement of dissent against psychiatry known as 'anti-psychiatry'.

Anti-Psychiatry

Although dissent against psychiatry had already been voiced before,[3] it was at the beginning of the 1960s that it gained unprecedented momentum, remaining a central concern throughout the 1970s. As Crossley (2006: 89) notes, referring to the British 'anti-psychiatrists':

---

3   For instance, in the United States in 1908, the former asylum inpatient Clifford Beers campaigned to improve the condition of asylum inmates (Beers, 1908). In the United Kingdom, in 1920, former inpatients established the *National Society for Lunacy Law Reform* for similar reasons (Fennell, 1996). In the 1920s the French playwright, theatre director, poet and actor Antonin Artaud gave voice, as a former asylum inmate, to a harsh criticism of institutional psychiatry, which, according to him, wished to impose reality and quash imagination (e.g., Artaud, 1947). In the 1950s, in the United States, protest against psychiatry came also from the right wing, who saw it as a pro-Communist endeavour that threatened individual rights. Such right-wing protesters grouped together against the Alaska Mental Health Bill – which allocated considerable funding for the improvement of Alaska inpatient psychiatric health care – and were joined by the Church of Scientology. Scientology's strong opposition to psychiatry has been often invoked to discredit the efforts of anti-psychiatry (e.g., Shorter, 1997: 282). See also Dain, 1989.

They infiltrated and to some degree 'colonised' the reading publics of the liberal and new left, becoming 'required reading' within its social circles, and were at the top reading lists for many university courses in the social sciences and humanities.

Such a remark could be easily extended beyond the British *milieu* to encompass the United States and Europe where, in the 1960s, protest against mainstream biological and institutional psychiatry was more and more widely discussed, in cultural circles and in academic environments, in psychiatric and medical journals as much as in left-wing magazines. Some of its exponents, such as R.D. Laing, became, to all effects and purposes, intellectual stars. This variegated and multifaceted wave of protest against psychiatry was called 'anti-psychiatry' by one of its foremost protagonists, David Cooper (1967), although most so-called 'anti-psychiatrists', such as Laing, Szasz and Basaglia himself, refused the label. We could argue that the foundations of this widespread challenge to psychiatry were laid between 1960 and 1961, with the almost simultaneous publication of a number of influential monographs: R.D. Laing's *The Divided Self* in 1960 and, in 1961, Michel Foucault's *Folie et déraison: Histoire de la folie à l'âge classique* (*History of Madness*), Erving Goffman's *Asylums: Essays on the Social Situation of Mental Patients and Other Inmates*, Frantz Fanon's *Les Damnés de la terre* (*The Wretched of the Earth*), and Thomas Szasz's *The Myth of Mental Illness*. All of these monographs consider psychiatry from a completely new perspective; namely, they clearly pinpoint the dependence of mainstream psychiatry on a historically produced and situated social order.

Heavily influenced by phenomeno-existentialist psychiatry, Laing (1990: 9) wrote *The Divided Self* with the aim of 'mak[ing] madness, and the process of going mad, comprehensible'. However, not unlike Basaglia in 'Il mondo dell'incomprensibile schizofrenico', Laing added an initial disclaimer to his preface: 'no attempt is made to present a comprehensive theory of schizophrenia. No attempt is made to explore constitutional and organic aspects' (Laing, 1990: 9). Initially, Laing's approach was not meant to challenge mainstream psychiatry, at least not entirely. However, three years later, in the 1964 preface to the Pelican edition of *The Divided Self* Laing was much less cautious:

> Psychiatry could be, and some psychiatrists are, on the side of transcendence, of genuine freedom, and of true human growth. But psychiatry can so easily be a technique of brainwashing, of inducing behaviour that is adjusted, by (preferably) non-injurious torture. In the best places, where straitjackets are abolished, doors are unlocked, leucotomies largely forgone, these can be replaced by more subtle lobotomies and tranquillizers that place the bars of Bedlam and the locked doors *inside* the patient. (Laing, 1990: 12)

The parallel with Basaglia is striking and it is not by chance that Basaglia delivered one of his most famous papers, 'La distruzione dell'ospedale psichiatrico', abandoning his initial caution and advocating the complete abolition of asylums, specifically during a conference on social psychiatry in London in 1964. In the same year, in 'What is Schizophrenia?', Laing (1964: 64) ironically refers to 'psychiatrosis', the syndrome of 'labelling others' using categories such as psychiatric diagnoses: schizophrenia is not a 'condition', he says, but a

> social fact. Indeed this label as social fact, is a political event. This political event, occurring in the civic order of society, imposes definitions and consequences on the labelled person. It is a social prescription that rationalizes a set of social actions whereby the labelled person is annexed by others, who are legally sanctioned, medically empowered, and morally obliged, to become responsible for the person labelled (Laing, 1964: 64).

Basaglia (1967b: 121) himself, explicitly drawing on Laing, does not hesitate to regard the psychiatric 'syndrome of labelling others' as a 'regressione nevrotica'.

All things considered, schizophrenia is, according to Laing (1964: 66), an 'explor[ation] of the inner space' that might well be 'one of the forms in which [...] the light beg[ins] to break through the cracks in our all-too-closed minds' (Laing, 1964: 68).

It was on these premises that, in 1965, the *Philadelphia Association*, founded two years earlier by Laing and Cooper among others, established the experimental therapeutic community[4] in Kingsley Hall, which rapidly

---

4   'Therapeutic Community' is a term coined by Thomas Main in his 1946 paper, 'The Hospital as a Therapeutic Institution', later developed and made famous by Maxwell

became 'the central hub for radicalism in the 1960s' (Crossley, 2006: 88). As Laing's son recalls, in Kingsley Hall,

> There were no 'patients', no 'doctors', no white coats, there was not 'mental illness', no 'schizophrenia' and therefore no 'schizophrenics' – just people living together. [...] There was a feeling of revolution about Kingsley Hall. The ideas and the people were so radical that the focal issues created the feeling that Kingsley Hall was a paradigm of psychiatric revolt, itself part of a wider, greater revolt, against the 'old order'. (Laing, 1997: 108)

For his part, Foucault was more interested in the specific historical evolution whereby the asylum eventually came to be entrusted with the containment of deviant behaviour. Starting with Philippe Pinel, whose act of freeing madmen from the chains in the *Salpêtrière* hospital is often considered to be the birth of modern psychiatry,[5] 'the asylum becomes

---

Jones. After World War II, Jones was appointed director of a social rehabilitation unit for disturbed prisoners-of-war. He involved the patients in community activities and tried to negotiate contacts with the external world (for instance with possible employers or former friends of the patients). In 1947, he became director of the Industrial Neurosis Unit (the future Social Rehabilitation Unit) in Belmont Hospital. He focused his research on the rehabilitation of chronic character disorders and developed the practice of 'social therapy'. It was Maxwell Jones who first structured the experience of a therapeutic community as an organic and official practice. Basaglia visited Jones's Dingleton Hospital in Scotland in 1961–62. From there, he imported the therapeutic community into his everyday practice in Gorizia's asylum. Elly Jansen claims that the therapeutic community 'should provide a communal living experience which encourages open communication, and promotes intrapsychic and social adjustment, to the maximum capacity of the individual' (Jansen, 1980: 32–33). Among the main principles of the meeting are the following: all participants must be present by agreement, the purpose of the meetings must be agreed beforehand by all participants, meeting is to obtain and give help, so that an inmate may eventually leave the community (Jansen, 1980: 24).

5   Philippe Pinel is considered to be the father of contemporary psychiatry. He is remembered for removing all forms of physical restraint (especially iron chains) from the *Hospice de la Salpêtrière*, and for his experiment with the so-called 'moral treatment'. When Pinel became the *Salpêtrière*'s director in 1795, the hospital was a huge village, where seven thousand destitute and sick women were interned. However,

[...] an instrument of moral uniformity and social denunciation' (Foucault, 2006a: 495). This instrument is:

> a form of social segregation [...] that guaranteed bourgeois morality a *de facto* universality, enabling it to impose itself as a system of law over all forms of alienation. (Foucault, 2006a: 495)

As Foucault put it, 'psychiatric practice is a certain moral tactic [...] covered over by the myths of positivism' (Foucault, 2006a: 509).

While Foucault focused on the historical evolution of the social mandate of institutional psychiatry, the sociologist Erving Goffman studied the contemporary condition of inmates inside the asylum, which he regarded as a 'total institution'. With this expression Goffman defines all those institutions, such as asylums, prisons or even schools and hospitals, which tend to encompass the life of inmates, controlling every single aspect of their existence. The 'total' character of the institution is reinforced by a 'barrier to social intercourse with the outside' (Goffman, 2007: 16), which divides the institution from everyday life. Inside this secluded space, the inmate experiences what Goffman calls a 'moral career'. This is a series of 'progressive changes', constantly monitored by the institution, 'that occur in the beliefs that [the inmate] has concerning himself and significant others' (Goffman, 2007: 24). Eventually, through this process, the inmate is deprived of his own self. The long-term effect of the 'moral career' is that the self of the inmate ceases to be:

> a property of the person to whom it is attributed but dwells rather in the pattern of social control that is exerted in connection with the person by himself and those around him. (Goffman, 2007: 154)

Pinel was not the first to remove physical restraint. At *Bicêtre*, where he worked before *Salpêtrière*, Pinel was under the supervision of the governor of the hospital, Jean-Baptiste Pussin, who was experimenting with what Pinel later called the 'moral treatment'. It consisted of a non-medical and non-violent approach to patients, which Pinel later applied at *Salpêtrière*. See Philippe Pinel, *Traité médico-philosophique sur l'aliénation mentale* (1800). Translated into English in 1806.

We have seen in the previous chapter the extent to which Basaglia agreed with Goffman about the notion of the institutionalised body. Indeed, *Asylums* was translated into Italian by Franca Ongaro and published by Einaudi with Basaglia's preface in 1968.

Goffman analyses the workings and effects of 'total institutions' from a sociological perspective. We have seen above that when these mechanisms are extended to states of domination such as colonialism the effects are devastating. In *The Wretched of the Earth*, Fanon proposed a controversial and much-debated solution to overcome this state of domination, a solution which was endorsed in the equally disputable introduction to the book written by Jean Paul Sartre. Fanon (1961: 37) suggests that a new world must come into being, and the only means of achieving this is through a total revolution, 'absolute violence'. To a certain extent, Basaglia was influenced by this position. As I will show in the next chapter, both Basaglia and Fanon believed that somehow the aggressiveness of the oppressed could be an answer to oppression itself. Furthermore, as Hopton (1995: 726) observed, Fanon reveals, within his analysis of the psychological effects of colonisation, that the relationship between the doctor and the patient is a 'microcosm of power relationships in wider society, and within oppressive societies mental institutions are places of coercion and not of healing'.

Finally, in his monograph, *The Myth of Mental Illness*, the psychiatrist Thomas Szasz questioned the existence of mental illness *tout court*. Szasz (2003: 1) goes so far as to affirm that 'there is no such thing as "mental illness"'. Szasz (1960) claims that 'the concept of illness, whether bodily or mental, implies deviation from some clearly defined norm'. Szasz was indebted to the work of the French philosopher and historian of sciences, George Canguilhem, in particular his 1943 *Essai sur quelques problèmes concernant le normal et le pathologique* (*The Normal and the Pathological*) in which he states (2007: 144) that 'there is no fact which is normal or pathological in itself'.[6] Whilst in physical medicine the norm can be ascribed to a certain integrity (whether functional or structural) (Szasz, 1960) or, as

---

6   Georges Canguilhem (1904–95) first published *Essai sur quelques problèmes concernant le normal et le pathologique* in 1943. This was republished in 1966 under the title

Canguilhem (2007: 197) puts it, to a 'margin of tolerance to the inconstancies of the environment', in the case of psychiatry, the norm is not so easily defined. Szasz (1960) maintains that this norm is 'stated in terms of psycho-social, ethical, and legal concepts'. Hence, while psychiatry claims to be a medical science, its distinction between health and illness is dictated by the dominant norms of society. I shall argue in the next chapter that Basaglia is especially sensitive to this theme. He claims that psychiatry is a means of perpetuating the dominant capitalist norm through the identification and seclusion of deviants under the guise of a medical science.

Michel Foucault

Michel Foucault played a key role in shaping and sustaining the challenge to psychiatry throughout the 1960s–1970s, thanks largely to the pioneering reach of his 1961 *History of Madness*, which was immediately regarded as one of the key works of 'anti-psychiatry'. Foucault's *History of Madness*, along with his later works on psychiatric power, and their impact on psychiatry and on Basaglia, are difficult to understand without contextualising them within Foucault's wider *oeuvre*. It is for this reason that over the next few sections I will detail the evolution of Foucault's analysis of madness, psychiatry and power, beginning with his initial interest in Binswanger's *Daseinanalyse* and phenomeno-existentialist psychiatry.

Foucault on Binswanger and Psychology

Michel Foucault is best known as a historian of systems of thought and as a philosopher but he began his career as a psychologist. During the late

---

Le Normal et le pathologique, augmenté de nouvelles réflexions concernant le normal et le pathologique.

1940s and early 1950s, he was mentored by Daniel Lagache and Georges Canguilhem; along with Jacques Lacan and Georges Daumézon, he attended Georges Gusdorf's lectures on psychopathology at the *École Normale*, and Henry Ey's presentations at the Saint Anne hospital, where he also worked as a psychology lab assistant. At the *Normale* and then at the Sorbonne, he attended Merleau-Ponty classes, where he met Ludwig Binswanger (Basso, 2007: 22). In 1954 Foucault published the introduction to the French translation of Binswanger's *Traum und Existenz* (*Dream and Existence*) (Foucault, 1984b) and his first monograph, *Maladie mentale et personnalité* (Foucault, 1954), which has never been translated into English.

These two publications sit somewhat oddly in Foucault's overall production, as May (2006) points out, in that Foucault later rejected phenomenology and the majority of his work – despite featuring a variety of methodological approaches – will always 'define itself *against* phenomenology' (May, 2006: 285). However, as Foucault himself later acknowledged, his first and short 'phenomenological phase' greatly contributed to his subsequent research, if anything because it allowed him to maintain a distance from the mainstream biological psychiatry he encountered as a psychologist, in order to begin analysing it from the archaeological and genealogical perspective we are familiar with:

> My reading of what was called 'existential analysis' or 'phenomenological psychiatry' was important for me during the time I was working in psychiatric hospitals and while I was looking for something different from the traditional schemas of psychiatric observation, a counterweight to them [...] existential analysis helped us to delimit and get a better grasp on what was heavy and oppressive in the gaze and the knowledge apparatus of academic psychiatry. (Foucault and Trombadori, 2001: 257–58)

In his introduction to Binswanger's work, Foucault focuses on the subjective experience of creating the world of dreams:

> The dream world is a world of its own, not in the sense of a subjective experience defying the norms of objectivity, but in the sense that it is constituted in the original mode of a world which belongs to me. (Foucault, 1984b: 51)

The subjective experience of creating the dream world ultimately epitomises the freedom of human beings:

> By reinstating the human subject in its radical freedom, the dream discloses paradoxically the movement of freedom toward the world, the point of origin from which freedom makes itself world. (Foucault, 1984b: 51)

Foucault is here concerned with the subjective modalities that construct the dream world and with the freedom that ultimately underpins human existence *tout court*.

The somewhat tortured editorial history of *Maladie mentale et personnalité*, instead, shows Foucault turning his attention to the study of mental illness from a much more critical standpoint. In 1962, Foucault published a completely revised edition of *Maladie mentale et personnalité*, entitled *Maladie mentale et psychologie*, subsequently translated into English and published under the title *Mental Illness and Psychology*.[7] However, neither version satisfied him: apparently, Foucault left a note expressly prohibiting all reprints of the 1954 version and he also tried, albeit unsuccessfully, to prevent the translation into English of the 1962 revised edition (Dreyfus, 1987: viii).[8] In *Maladie mentale et personnalité* Foucault focuses mainly on the phenomeno-existential study of the psychology of mental illness. *Mental Illness and Psychology*, published a year after *History of Madness*, features a second part,[9] entitled *Madness and Culture* (Foucault, 1987:

---

7   I shall henceforth refer to this work and the parts of it by their English titles.
8   According to Foucault, *Mental Illness and Psychology* (Foucault, 1987) left him dissatisfied for two main reasons. In the first draft of the introduction to the second volume of *History of Sexuality* he acknowledged, on the one hand, a 'theoretical weakness in elaborating the notion of experience' but on the other hand, he also regarded his treatment of psychiatry as an 'ambiguous link [...] simultaneously ignored and taken for granted' (Foucault, 1984a: 334).
9   In the 1954 version, the second part – *The Actual Conditions of Illness* – advanced 'a Marxist account of mental illness and a Pavlovian account of its organic basis' (Dreyfus, 1987: viii). This version was completely replaced by the 1962 Part II. Dreyfus believes that the main weakness of *Maladie mentale et personnalité* was precisely its 'unstable combination of Heideggerian existential anthropology and Marxist social history' (Dreyfus, 1987: viii). Shortly before his death, in an interview with Charles

59–85), which amounts to a summary of the conclusions drawn in *History of Madness*. The first part of *Mental Illness and Psychology* (Foucault, 1987: 15–84), which is the same in the two versions of the monograph, relates notably to Basaglia's early philosophical approach to psychiatry: both Foucault and Basaglia insisted on the centrality of phenomenological 'understanding' as a proper method of investigating mental illness and both also stressed the importance of the body as a medium for the self to relate to the world. However, the second part, added in 1962, does not contribute much to the conclusions Foucault reaches in *History of Madness*, on which I shall therefore focus my attention in the following section.

Foucault's Graft

History of Madness is a multifaceted work; as Khalfa (2006) observes in his introduction to the English edition, it has at least three possible readings. First of all, it is a history of the process that brought about the medicalisation of madness. Secondly, as Foucault himself claims, the aim of *History of Madness* is to unravel why and when human beings became possible subjects of psychological research. Khalfa (2006: xix) sees in this Foucault's first definition of the 'particular brand of historiography that he named, in this book, the "archeology of knowledge"'.[10] Finally, it marks Foucault's

---

Ruas, the translator of *Death and the Labyrinth*, Foucault himself expressed reservations about his use of existential analysis, phenomenology and Marxism: 'I was divided between existential psychology and phenomenology, and my research was an attempt to discover the extent these could be defined in historical terms. That's when I first understood that the subject would have to be defined in other terms than Marxism or phenomenology' (Foucault and Ruas, 2004: 176–77).

10 Foucault (2002b) expanded the concept of the 'archeology of knowledge' in the text of the same name. The archeology of knowledge is very different from a history of ideas, which is 'the discipline of beginning and ends, the description of [...] continuities and returns, the reconstruction of developments in the linear form of history'. A history of ideas focuses on retrieving the 'genesis, continuity and totalisation' (Foucault, 2002b: 154) of history. The archeology of knowledge, on the other hand, is not 'an interpretative discipline'; that is to say, it does not look at historical

shift from phenomenological research to a structuralist approach; while Foucault still refers to the horizon of subjective experience, he does so in order to structure such experiences under the articulation of norms and principles. The aim of this history is to unravel how the transformation of such norms bears witness to the changing structures that produce them.

Although *History of Madness* can be read from many different perspectives, it has been subjected to unambiguous criticism. The main critique levelled against it is that Foucault does not sufficiently support his argument with consistent historical data. For instance, Scull (1990: 57) believes that while *History of Madness* 'is a provocative and dazzling [...] poem', it also rests on the 'shakiest of scholarly foundations', and Midelfort (1980: 259) states that many of *History of Madness*'s arguments 'fly in the face of empirical evidence, and that many of its broadest generalizations are oversimplifications'. Many other scholars share the same reservations (for instance, Sedgwick, 1982: 131–32; Hacking, 1986: 29; LaCapra, 1990: 32–34). This criticism legitimately problematises the historical data that endorse Foucault's main argument. Nevertheless, I also believe that, as Gutting (2005: 50) puts it, *History of Madness* should be primarily praised for its 'meta-level claims about how madness should be approached as a historiographical topic'. That is to say, the importance of *History of Madness* lies not so much in the historical data it presents as in its study of the changes throughout history to the concept of madness.

Although *History of Madness* can be regarded as a history of the representation of madness, it should not be considered as a history of

---

> data and documents to find a 'better-hidden discourse'. Rather, it seeks to reconstruct how specific discourses became 'practices obeying certain rules' (Foucault, 2002b: 155). If we take the example of HM, an archeology of the discourse on madness, we can see how Foucault does not try to find the 'innermost secret of the origin' (2002b: 156) of this discourse, nor does he try to transform its evolution into a continuity. Instead, Foucault is 'rewriting' the history of madness; that is, he focuses on 'the preserved form of exteriority', i.e. the representation of madness through the centuries, in order to produce a 'regulated transformation of what has already been written'. In other words, Foucault (2002b: 156) is advancing a 'systematic description of the discourse' on madness.

psychiatry. As Still and Velody (1992: 4) observe, this book is a 'history of the significance of madness', which may not have a direct connection with the 'disciplinary history of how specially trained professionals dealt with it'. In any case, its first appearance in English[11] greatly influenced the 'anti-psychiatric' movement. In Armstrong's words (1997: 16), the abridged edition of *History of Madness* 'was rapidly recruited to the anti-psychiatry side'. Despite the fact that *History of Madness*'s main focus is the representation of madness rather than that of psychiatry, it represented a challenge to mainstream biological psychiatrists insofar as it showed 'that the practitioner does not know his subjects as well as he thinks' (Barham, 1992: 49). Unfolding the history of madness was soon considered to be a 'method which allowed one to put brackets round medical rationalizations' (Castel, 1992: 66). Castel goes so far as to maintain that, with *History of Madness*, madness became a 'kernel of authenticity', that is, the paradigm of a free subject (Castel, 1992: 67). Indeed, a number of anti-psychiatrists reached such a radical conclusion (for example, Laing saw schizophrenia as an inner voyage), also drawing on Foucault. It is not necessary, though, to reach such radical conclusions in recognising the centrality of *History of Madness* for the psychiatric practitioner: it shook the scientific foundations of psychiatry mainly because it revealed that mental illness is a 'variable social construct, not an ahistorical scientific given' (Gutting, 2005: 50).

The history of madness can be roughly divided into three ages (Khalfa, 2006: xv), the first being the Renaissance, when the discourse on madness became a 'reflection on wisdom'. After this came the Classical age (the seventeenth and eighteenth centuries), during which the 'institutions of confinement' were born. In these, madmen were interned along with the destitute, the poor and the sick. Finally, the 'modern experience of madness'

---

11   *Histoire de la folie à l'âge classique* appeared in English for the first time in 1965. This translation is based on the abridged French edition (*Folie et Déraison*), and bears the title of *Madness and Civilization*. It consists of less than half of the original, the abridgement amounting to over three hundred of the five hundred pages, most of the footnotes and all of the bibliography. The unabridged edition was not translated into English and published (by Routledge) until 2006, although its introduction appeared in 2002 in *Pli* (Foucault, 2002a).

came into being with the creation of the asylum, i.e. a special institution dedicated to the treatment of madmen. In the age of the asylum, madness was to be perceived as the object of positive sciences, to be studied as an object and treated as an illness. It was at this point, at the beginning of the age of the asylum, that an important concept emerged in Foucault's discourse: that of the 'graft'.

> For this new reason which reigns in the asylum – says Foucault – madness does not represent the absolute form of contradiction but instead a minority status, an aspect of itself that does not have the right to autonomy, and can live only *grafted* onto the world of reason [added emphasis]. (Foucault, 2006a: 489)

The reason why Foucault relies on the practice of grafting to describe the relationship between madness and reason can be traced back to its common meaning: in botany, different plants can be grafted to form new hybrids. According to the *Dictionary of Plant Sciences*, the definition of 'to graft' in botany is:

> to transfer a part of an organism from its normal position to another position on the same organism (autograft), or to a different organism of the same species (homograft), or an organism of a different species (heterograft). (Allaby, 2006)

Suffice it to say that, although two different entities can be combined to form a new one, the relationship between the two plants is *not equal*: if plant A is grafted onto plant B, it is the latter that provides the new AB hybrid with what it needs to survive (nutrition, water, etc.). When we extend the practice of grafting from botany to a conceptual and metaphorical level, an important implication emerges. If, in botany, a graft is mainly a transfer and a creation, on a conceptual level it is also, and possibly above all, a relation of power.

When Foucault describes madness as a graft onto the world of reason, his use of the term 'graft' highlights the inequality between the two elements rather than their fusion or, to put it in another way, it defines the fusion between them in terms of their original inequality. For it to participate in the totality of the social body madness must first be marked as different, separated, stigmatised and then grafted onto reason, from which, like a grafted plant, it derives all its sustenance. In other words, madness is conceptualised as being radically different from reason yet subordinate to it, a state of affairs the origins of which Foucault places with Descartes. Foucault (2006a: 45) accuses Descartes of concluding, in his *First Meditation*, that 'madness is precisely a condition of impossibility for thought' and therefore that it is 'simply excluded by the doubting subject, in the same manner that it will soon be excluded that he is not thinking or that he does not exist'. Ultimately, in Descartes,

> the perils of madness have been quashed by the exercise of Reason, and this new sovereign rules a domain where the only possible enemies are errors and illusions. The process of Descartes' doubt breaks the spells woven by the senses and steers a clear course through the landscape of dreams, constantly guided by the light of true things. But madness is banished in the name of the man who doubts, and who is no more capable of opening himself to unreason than he is of not thinking or not being. (Foucault, 2006a: 46)

Foucault's accusations were challenged, some years after the publication of *History of Madness*, by Jacques Derrida (2001), in his 1963 paper 'Cogito and the History of Madness', where he contended that Descartes had not been as dismissive of madness as Foucault made it seem. To dwell on the debate would be to steer the argument off topic; therefore, suffice it to say that Derrida's paper sparked a heated and influential debate that continued in Foucault's papers 'My Body, This Paper, This Fire' and 'Reply to Derrida' (published as Appendix II and III respectively of the 1972 French edition of *History of Madness*, and translated into English in 2006).[12]

Overall, Foucault's entire reflection on psychiatric power can be seen as an archeological interest in the graft between madness and reason. On the one hand, he studies diachronically how such a graft was established, how it came into being. On the other hand, he carries out a synchronic analysis of how psychiatry as it was practised in the 1960s was only the most recent incarnation of this graft, and thus it had a precise history – it was not, that is, based on an ahistorical scientific paradigm.

12   On the debate between Foucault and Derrida see, for example, Boyne, 1990; D'Amico, 1984; Flaherty 1986; Cook 1990.

On a diachronic level, when the first graft was established between madness and reason, it renewed a form of repression and exclusion that was once associated with lepers. In Foucault's words (2006a: 52), 'the empty space left by the disappearance of leprosy was now peopled with new characters'. During what Foucault refers to as the era of the 'great confinement', madmen were indiscriminately associated with criminals, the poor and the destitute. Confinement was an 'economic measure and a social precaution' that constituted a 'determining factor in the experience of madness'. In fact, in its association with poverty and indigence, madness came to be recognised as 'one of the problems of the city' (Foucault, 2006a: 77).

When, at the end of the eighteenth century, Philippe Pinel freed madmen from the chains of the 'great confinement' and established the moral treatment, madness was to be hidden away in a more sophisticated and specific place. As a consequence of these processes of 'excommunication', madness eventually became 'an object of knowledge' (Foucault, 2006a: 104). According to Foucault, this happened precisely when madness was transformed into mental illness. Yet, while the asylum was represented as 'a free domain of observation, diagnosis and therapeutics' of mental illnesses, it turned out to be nothing less than a 'judicial space where people were accused, judged and sentenced'. Foucault's assertion (2006a: 503) is unequivocal: 'For a long time to come, and at least until today, [madness] was imprisoned in a moral world'. The link between morality and medicine came into being through the fear that the disregard that madmen showed for decency – or their outright immorality – could be contagious. In Foucault's words (2006a: 355), 'people were in dread of a [...] sickness that [...] emanated from the houses of confinement'. This fear shaped for the first time the link between madness and reason in medical terms: madness 'found itself facing medical thought' (Foucault, 2006a: 358).

According to Gutting, the main argument of *History of Madness* revolves precisely around this point: this book 'is intended as a basis for showing that madness as mental illness was a social construction [...] original with the nineteenth century' (Gutting, 2005: 53). The primary characteristic of the newly discovered mental illness was not, as one might expect from an illness, a specific set of medical symptoms; rather, it amounted to a certain distance from rationality. In *History of Madness*, Foucault maintained that this rationality consisted of the acceptable standards of bourgeois society, an argument that would prove central to 'anti-psychiatry' and to Basaglia. That is to say, mental illness was not so much a medical condition as 'the stigma of a class that had abandoned the forms of bourgeois ethics' (Foucault, 2006a: 378). Mental illness became 'the most immediate threat' to the bourgeois order (Foucault, 2006a: 379). The encapsulating of madness in the concept of mental illness turned madmen into social outcasts and a threat to society: madmen were simply defined as such by the ruling class through reference to behaviour which seemed to oppose its moral dictates. The humanitarian act of dividing the sick from the criminals and freeing them from chains became 'not the liberation of unreason but madness mastered in advance' (Foucault, 2006a: 489). Madmen became 'sick' precisely when they began to embody the intersection of a 'legally irresponsible subject and a man who troubled the social [bourgeois] order' (Foucault, 2006a: 128). As Basaglia (1967d: 145) put it,

> Quando Pinel liberò i folli dalle prigioni, separandoli dal delinquente e restituendo loro la dignità della malattia di cui soffrivano, non ha fatto altro che spostarli in una nuova prigione in cui l'inferiorità morale del recluso era scientificamente sancita, e la reclusione scientificamente giustificata. Ciò senza che l'atteggiamento generale della società nei confronti del folle mutasse minimamente, né il tipo di rapporto, né la distanza che lo separa dagli altri.

Madness 'was never *made manifest* on its own terms', excluded as it was from society on the one hand, and made the object of a medical science on the other. Rather, it continued to be split 'between the two terms of the dichotomy' (Foucault, 2006a: 171), between medicine and morality, objectification and exclusion. Through these conceptualisations, the product of the age of the asylum was a specific space (both physical and conceptual) which could incarnate the graft between madness and reason that Foucault theorised.

In *History of Madness*, Foucault referred for the first time to the concept of 'graft' in relation to madness and reason. More specifically, *History of Madness* could be read as the history of the graft between madness and reason: while the conception of the graft properly emerged only after the 'great confinement', we can see it evolving throughout *History of Madness*, until finally it gains a definitive shape in the modern asylum. I believe that the concept of graft persists in Foucault's thought, and that his entire reflection on psychiatric power could be read as an articulation of it. In the following section, I analyse the two main characteristics of psychiatric power: discipline and normalisation. I believe that the following considerations should not only be regarded as a historical description of how the graft between madness and reason came into being and evolved during the modern era; they also show how the graft is maintained and regulated by the psychiatry which Basaglia so strongly criticised.

Disciplinary Psychiatry

Both in the 1973–74 course *Psychiatric Power* (Foucault, 2006b) and in the 1975 monograph *Discipline and Punish* (Foucault, 1991), Foucault describes what he calls 'disciplinary power'. In the latter, Foucault defines 'discipline' as 'a type of power [...] comprising a whole set of instruments, techniques, procedures, levels of application, targets' that 'may be taken over by "specialised" institutions' in order to 'reinforc[e] or reorganiz[e] their internal mechanisms of power' (Foucault, 1991: 215). In other words, disciplinary power is composed of a number of techniques that can be 'totally appropriated in certain institutions' (Dreyfus and Rabinow, 1982: 153) such as schools, prisons or asylums. Although *Discipline and Punish* is the primary reference for understanding disciplinary power in Foucault, I will refer mostly to *Psychiatric Power* because it focuses more closely on the evolution of psychiatry into its mainstream biological and institutional form.

According to Foucault (2006b: 40), discipline is what enables political power to reach 'the level of bodies and to get hold of them', with the aim of producing a 'human being who could be treated as a docile [and productive] body' (Dreyfus and Rabinow, 1982: 134–35). From a diachronic perspective,[13] disciplinary power is preceded by sovereign power, which

---

13   For the sake of clarity and for the time being, I will assume that disciplinary power follows sovereign power in a chronological order, leaving a more detailed

establishes an asymmetrical 'link between sovereign and subject' (Foucault, 2006b: 42). In a relationship of sovereignty, the centre of power, the sovereign, imposes levies and taxes on the subjects without having to give them anything in return – 'for the sovereign does not have to pay back' (Foucault, 2006b: 42). There is thus a wide dissymmetry between the one who exerts power, the sovereign, who receives and does not have to give anything in return, and the ones over whom power is exerted, the subjects, who give in order to receive nothing. Despite this dissymmetry, sovereign power can only partially get hold of individuals; for instance, it seizes a part of the goods of the individual through a tax, when it threatens them with torture, or when it celebrates the power of the sovereign in a ceremony. Contrary to this, disciplinary power 'is a seizure of the body, [...] of time in its totality' (Foucault, 2006b: 46). In a relationship of sovereignty, the sovereign exerts power *discontinuously*, for instance when he needs to obtain a tax from his subjects. The disciplinary seizure of the body, on the other hand, entails an exertion of power which is not fragmented. Because discipline aims at creating a 'docile body' that 'may be subjected, used, transformed and improved' (Foucault, 1991: 136), it calls for a total and continuous control. This continuity is encapsulated in the idea that the body should be disciplined with constant exercise. The effectiveness of these exercises is assessed by a plethora of teachers, supervisors, assistants, who are constantly ready to intervene. This constant visibility establishes what Foucault (2006b: 52) defined as the 'panoptic character of disciplinary power', around which the argument of *Discipline and Punish* revolves.

The concept of 'panopticism' originates with Jeremy Bentham's utopian prison, the *Panopticon* (1838). This was a circular structure that had the inmates' cells on the external perimeter, while the superintendent was located at the centre. While he could see all that was happening in the cells, the inmates could never see the central surveillance process. As Foucault (1991: 201) says, the *Panopticon* induces 'in the inmate a state of conscious and permanent visibility that assures the automatic functioning of power'.

---

discussion of Foucault's oscillations between sovereignty, discipline, and biopolitics for Chapter 5.

In Bertani's (2004: 64) words, the *Panopticon* fulfils a 'principio di visibilità permanente'. According to Foucault, this is the utopia of disciplinary power: to achieve the total visibility of all individuals, without exposing the source of power.

Disciplinary systems work on a double mechanism: on the one hand, they are 'normalising' insofar as they establish a criterion of normality – 'an average to be respected or [...] an optimum towards which one must move' (Foucault, 1991: 183) – and also a series of exercises (Foucault, 2006b: 54) to make individuals reach this condition. On the other hand, disciplines are 'anomising'; that is to say, they continuously discard those individuals who cannot be normalised. This is the reason why discipline necessarily entails a margin, insofar as not all individuals might be disciplined effectively. This mechanism is not at work in a relationship of sovereignty as the latter 'applies [...] to multiplicities [...] which are in a way situated above physical individuality' (Foucault, 2006b: 44). For this reason, discipline inverts the so-called pyramid of power that is at work in sovereignty. There is 'an elimination of individualization at the top'; that is, there is no sovereign, while there is 'a very strong underlying individualization at the base' (Foucault, 2006b: 55). In other words, discipline stems from an unidentifiable source in order to exert power not on a multitude but on every single individual; it is 'invisible and dispersed' (Smith, 2000: 290). Disciplinary power literally creates the individual, as it produces 'new gestures, actions, habits, and skills, and ultimately new kinds of people' (Rouse, 2005: 98).

This is why Foucault believes that the individual does not pre-exist discipline. As Elden (2006: 49) puts it, the very 'constitution of the individual is a product of a certain technology of power, namely discipline'. Foucault (2006b: 56) maintains that 'what we should call the individual is the effect produced on the somatic singularity', which derives from disciplinary techniques. The individual is an effect of power, 'a subjected body held in a system of supervision and subjected to procedures of normalization' (Foucault, 2006b: 57). Since its emergence, disciplinary power has, in fact, been 'concerned not with repressing but with creating' (Armstrong, 1995: 23). To be more specific, discipline creates the individual, which is as such always-already woven into relations of power. The modern acceptation of 'human being' as such is an 'after-image', resulting from 'the technology employed by the [...] bourgeoisie to constitute the individual in the field of productive and political forces' – i.e. discipline (Foucault, 2006b: 58). To put it simply, modern human beings are, according to Foucault, individuals who are themselves the product of the domination of the bourgeoisie.

How does such a conceptualisation of discipline apply to psychiatry? It could be said that, according to Foucault, psychiatry is not only the discipline of the *undisciplined* but also the *discipline of disciplines*. We have seen that disciplinary systems always have a margin, made of those who cannot be normalised. It is in this margin that psychiatry begins to operate, when it takes on itself the 'role of discipline for all those who could not be disciplined' (Foucault, 2006b: 86). Foucault is somewhat unclear with regard to the history that led psychiatry to becoming the discipline of disciplines. According to him, the person who was 'inassimilable, incapable of being disciplined, or uneducable' (Foucault, 2006b: 81) was sent back to his own family, who had the role of 'rejecting him in turn [and] getting rid of him' (Foucault, 2006b: 82). When, at the end of this process, the family rejected the abnormal person, 'he was put in a psychiatric hospital' (Foucault, 2006b: 85). This is why Elden (2006: 50) affirms that the family had 'a crucial role in fixing individuals into disciplinary systems'. When all disciplinary apparatuses (such as the school, the army, the workshop, etc.) failed, and when the family also failed, psychiatry 'stepped in' (Foucault, 2006b: 86) and compensated for these failures. Basaglia (1967d: 146) very much agreed with Foucault on this point:

> Il nostro sistema familiare e sociale sembra specializzato nell'individuazione precoce (quando addirittura non si tratta di creazione) di deboli, sui quali concentrare l'aggressività di tutti. Quasi ogni gruppo familiare ha il suo capro espiatorio che, qualche volta, finisce in manicomio come 'uomo di troppo'. E il manicomio, allora, si affretta a sancire scientificamente il suo significato di 'eccedenza', rifiutandogli anche la parvenza di un ruolo e riducendolo a pura oggettività.

In these ways, psychiatry became the discipline that could establish all the 'schemas for the individualization, normalization, and subjection of individuals within disciplinary systems' (Foucault, 2006b: 86).

Upon admission to the asylum – or, to use Goffman's terms, at the beginning of their moral career – patients/inmates undergo four impositions. The first is the imposition of the 'other': the person who is mentally ill has to accept otherness as a 'source of power', to which one 'must be subjugated' (Foucault, 2006b: 176). The second imposition is identity: upon admission to the asylum and other institutions, inmates must state their name and other biographical details. According to Foucault, this should confine the inmate inside 'his own history', because he must recognise himself in an 'identity constituted by certain episodes in his life' (2006b: 159). The patient is then subjected to the 'reality of illness itself'; that is, psychiatric intervention is always about 'showing the mad person that his madness is madness and that he really is ill' (Foucault, 2006b: 176). The patient must perceive himself as sick; he must believe he is ill. Additionally, he is required to alienate himself completely into the diagnosis. As Laing (1990: 34) points out, 'no one has schizophrenia, like having a cold [...] he is schizophrenic'. This is why Roberts (2005: 38) rightly stresses that

> in being 'invited' to understand themselves accordingly, and in being understood as such by others, [the patients are] 'tied' to a specific identity through a 'conscience or self-knowledge'.

Finally, the patient must accept 'everything corresponding to the techniques concerning money'; that is to say, the dimension of 'need', and the fact that one must work, earn, and exchange these earnings with services to 'provide for [one's] needs' (Foucault, 2006b: 177).

So far though, there is little in its history that tells us why madness became the domain of medicine with the creation of a specialty for mental illness, i.e. psychiatry. In *History of Madness*, Foucault (2006a: 508) had already considered the process that led to psychiatry becoming a branch of medicine nothing short of a 'dense mystery'; in fact, 'as positivism imposed itself [...] on psychiatry, the practice became more obscure, the power of the psychiatrist more miraculous' (2006a: 508). According to Foucault, the medical nature of psychiatry is at the very least questionable. In this regard, he poses the following question in *Psychiatric Power*: 'What medical practice inhabits [the asylum]?' (Foucault, 2006b: 129). He gives a twofold answer. On the one hand, it is the nosological discourse, the description and classification of the various manifestations of madness into different mental illnesses and syndromes; a discourse that serves only as a 'sort of *analogon* of medical truth'. On the other, it is the anatomo-pathological knowledge, which researches the 'organic correlatives of madness', and which serves as 'the materialist guarantee of psychiatric practice' (Foucault, 2006b: 133). Both discourses are only 'guarantees of truth' (Foucault, 2006b: 134) and are never really put to work in the asylum.

Normality and Abnormality

These considerations primarily concern psychiatry as it was practised in the asylum, the public psychiatric hospital of the nineteenth century. Yet, as Beaulieu rightly points out, the evolution of disciplinary power brought about a change. By the beginning of the twentieth century, psychiatric power no longer aimed 'to proliferate within institutions but rather to break out of institutions' (Beaulieu, 2006: 27), as part of the widespread process that Foucault (1991: 216) called the 'formation of disciplinary society',[14] which required that disciplinary power escaped from the enclosed institutions where it originated. In disciplinary society the 'effects of power' can be brought to the most 'minute and distant elements', in that discipline 'assures an infinitesimal distribution of power relations' (Foucault, 1991: 216). From the 1840s and through to the 1860s, psychiatrists began to stress the importance of showing the intrinsic dangerousness of madmen, even if this entailed writing false reports. It was as if they felt the need to 'transform an act of assistance into a phenomenon of protection' (Foucault, 2006b: 220). Since this could not be based on a true medical practice, because of its 'mancanza di un corpo anatomico' (Colucci, 2006b: 176), psychiatry became a form of preventive social defence.

---

14   It is unclear in *Discipline and Punish* whether Foucault regards 'disciplinary society' as a stage that chronologically follows the rise of discipline in enclosed institutions. I will return to this in Chapter 5.

This was made possible through a 'psychiatrization of the child' (Foucault, 2006b: 203). Psychiatrists began to look for early manifestations of a possible future dangerousness and they looked for this predisposition in childhood. The abnormal child, and abnormality in general, became the condition that precedes madness. In this way, psychiatrists seized power not just over madmen but 'over the abnormal' (Foucault, 2006b: 221), insofar as every abnormal individual 'is a possible criminal' (Foucault, 2006b: 250).[15]

'Abnormal' is precisely the title of the course at the *Collège de France* that followed *Psychiatric Power*. In this course, Foucault explored how psychiatry became involved with law and justice, and how this effectively extended the influence of psychiatry into daily life. Psychiatrists were first asked, in criminal cases, to give an expert opinion as to whether the defendant were suffering from a mental illness, on the grounds of which one could plead extenuating circumstances. In this way psychiatry took the form of an *expertise*, through which psychiatrists were able to suggest the 'point of origin and the site where [the crime] took shape' (Foucault, 2003a: 17), and to show 'how the individual already resembles the crime before he has committed it' (Foucault, 2003a: 19) – of particular importance in this regard was the work of the Italian Cesare Lombroso[16] – as this resem-

---

15 Foucault's interest in the intersection between psychiatry and justice precedes the course *Abnormal*. In 1973, Foucault had edited and published the memoirs of the parricide Pierre Rivière, along with other documents concerning the case, such as the psychiatric expertises (translated into English in 1978). The case, dating back to 1836, bears witness to the process that Foucault describes in *Abnormal*. In his own words, the collection of documents on Pierre Rivière 'provided the intersection of discourses that differed in origin, form, organisation and function [...] in their totality and their variety they form neither a composite work nor an exemplary text but rather a strange contest, a confrontation, a power relation' (Foucault, 1978: x).

16 In his 1876 book *L'uomo delinquente*, the alienist Cesare Lombroso (1835–1909) argued that the born criminal, the atavistic criminal, could be identified by a certain number of physical traits, or stigmas, such as an asymmetrical face, abnormal eyes, excessive dimension of the jaw and cheek bones, protruding lips, abundance of wrinkles, supernumerary fingers, etc. Lombroso wanted to create an objective and scientific criminal anthropology, grounded on the measurement of physical traits

blance is already manifest in childhood.[17] In Foucault's words (2003a: 302), one can identify the condition of psychiatrisation 'inasmuch as the adult resembles what he was as a child, [...] inasmuch as one can rediscover an earlier wickedness in today's act'. Psychiatry thus brought about the belief that the kernel of possible dangerousness is 'endemic in the population', as opposed to the 'old insanity, which was restricted to the unfortunate few' (Armstrong, 1995: 25). Through this recognition, psychiatry began to function as 'public hygiene' (Foucault, 2003a: 119), by being, on the one hand, the negative technique of preventing crime and, on the other, the 'positive technique of intervention and transformation, a sort of normative project' (Foucault, 2003a: 50). The moment in which 'psychiatry "disalienizes" itself' (Foucault, 2003a: 160) is what Foucault (2003a: 121) refers to as the 'enthronement of psychiatry'. That is to say, psychiatry shifts its sphere of intervention from madmen, i.e. aliens, to children and addresses their possible abnormality as a sign of a future illness/dangerousness. Psychiatry effectively steps out from behind the walls of the asylum to become the

---

  of individuals and comparing them through the statistical analysis of the population. In order to understand the natural determinism of the criminal, 'meglio [...] abbandonare [...] le sublimi regioni delle teorie filosofiche, [...] e procedere invece allo studio diretto, somatico e psichico, dell'uomo criminale, confrontandolo colle risultanze offerte dall'uomo sano e dall'alicnato' (Lombroso, 1896: xxxiv–xxxv).

17 Despite such a focus on childhood, this assumption is very different from the psychoanalytic idea that neuroses originate in repressed childhood memories, which Freud formulated as early as 1895 in his *Studies on Hysteria*: 'Events from childhood establish a symptom of varying degrees of severity which persists for many years to come' (Freud and Breuer, 1895: 8). Foucault is describing a process through which the very biological nature of the human being is put at stake: psychiatrists are to find in childhood the organic characteristics of potential abnormality, i.e. the sign of a potential danger, in order to prevent it. The child is psychiatrised before the adult. On the contrary, in psychoanalysis there is no preventive aim. It is from the standpoint of the adult that childhood is addressed as the repository of those memories – often regarded as 'trivial and unimportant matters' (Freud, 1901: 45) – that can unravel the aetiology of the neurosis. While abnormal psychiatry targets the child before he can become a dangerous adult, psychoanalysis targets the remnants of childhood in the neurotic (and normal) adult.

knowledge entrusted with the definition of normality and the discipline entrusted with the renormalisation of abnormal people.

Foucault's and Basaglia's views as to the ultimate outcome of such a psychiatry – we might call it 'disciplinary psychiatry' – be it practised inside or outside of the asylum would eventually converge. As I discuss at length in the next chapter, Basaglia believed that psychiatric patients are deviants rather than merely sick, 'individui che per motivi diversi non partecipano alla produzione' (Basaglia and Ongaro Basaglia, 1971: 176). According to Foucault (2006b: 112), the aim of psychiatry is precisely to 'take out of circulation individuals who cannot be employed in the apparatus of production [so as to be] turned into a new source of profit'. This is another way of stating, in economic terms, the principle that Foucault had already expressed in *History of Madness*, namely that madness came to be perceived as a threat to bourgeois society.

On the basis of this analysis of the courses *Psychiatric Power* and *Abnormal*, I believe that it is possible to see how Foucault was returning to the concept of 'graft'. In summarising the disciplinary character of psychiatry, Foucault says that, all things considered, the truth produced by psychiatry 'is not the truth of madness speaking in its own name but the truth of a madness agreeing to first person recognition of itself in a particular administrative and medical reality' (Foucault, 2006b: 161). Esposito (2007: 172) follows on from Foucault's argument and states that madmen, along with other 'vite misere, anguste, [...] scellerate',

> non avendo mai giocato un ruolo soggettivo di primo piano, sfuggendo, per così dire, alle maglie della storia e perdendosi nell'anonimato dell'esistenza, non ci parlano mai in prima persona, non pronunciano mai il pronome 'io', né si rivolgono mai a un 'tu'. Non sono altro che dei fatti, o degli eventi, in terza persona.

In other words, the discourse *of* madness was never permitted; rather, a discourse *on* madness was produced through disciplinary psychiatry. This discourse forced madness to continue being a 'graft' onto the world of reason, inasmuch as there is a science that studies madness, classifies it as an illness, spots its early (alleged) manifestations, and treats it accordingly. Thus, psychiatry becomes the knowledge that can enforce, maintain, and regulate this graft, all the more so as it leaves the asylum to extend its gaze into the everyday life of individuals. These considerations converge with what Basaglia (1979c: 5) writes in a recently published posthumous essay:

> per noi la follia [...] è una cosa seria. La malattia mentale è invece il vuoto [...] la costruzione [...] per tenere celata, nascosta l'irrazionalità. Chi può parlare è solo la Ragione, la ragione del più forte, la ragione dello Stato e mai quella del diseredato, dell'emarginato, di chi non ha.

Like Foucault, according to Basaglia 'Reason' imposes a certain discourse on madness, in order to keep the needs of what he calls the subaltern class concealed. With this in mind, after this excursus on the main exponents of the 1960s criticism of psychiatry, with a special focus on Foucault's work, in the following chapter I return to the work of Franco Basaglia.

CHAPTER 4

'The Destruction of the Asylum'

Introduction

During a famous series of conferences in Brazil, in 1979, Franco Basaglia delivered a number of papers discussing the work of deinstitutionalisation he had carried out in Italy. During the second conference, in São Paulo (19 June 1979), Basaglia was asked if psychiatric intervention was possible at all without an institution to back it. Basaglia did not directly answer the question but took the opportunity to state:

> Non so cosa sia la follia. Può essere tutto o niente. È una condizione umana. In noi la follia esiste ed è presente come lo è la ragione. Il problema è che la società, per dirsi civile, dovrebbe accettare tanto la ragione quanto la follia. Invece questa società riconosce la follia come parte della ragione, e la riduce alla ragione nel momento in cui esiste una scienza che si incarica di eliminarla. Il manicomio ha la sua ragione di essere, perché fa diventare razionale l'irrazionale. Quando qualcuno è folle ed entra in un manicomio, smette di essere folle per trasformarsi in malato. Il problema è come sciogliere questo nodo, superare la follia istituzionale e riconoscere la follia là dove essa ha origine: nella vita. (Basaglia, 2000: 34)

It seems clear from this statement that Basaglia, when assessing *a posteriori* the work of deinstitutionalisation, believed that psychiatry intertwines madness and reason. It weaves them together inasmuch as it defines madness as something to be rationalised and thus makes it possible for it to be reintegrated into reason. Reforming psychiatry therefore means undoing this *nodo*; in other words, understanding madness not in rationalising medical terms as a mental illness but as a human condition. The concept of the *nodo* [knot/tangle] is remarkably close to Foucault's idea of the graft. In the previous chapter, I discussed how, according to Foucault, this graft was born and how it functions through disciplinary power. It is now time to understand the way in which Basaglia's *nodo* works and, especially, how Basaglia sets out to undo this knot.

Establishing a link between Basaglia's *nodo* and Foucault's graft endorses Di Vittorio's claim (1999: 111) that 'una verità storica può dimostrarsi strategicamente efficace'. In his monograph, *Foucault e Basaglia*, Di Vittorio advances the idea that Basaglia's work of deinstitutionalisation could and should be regarded as the 'practical' outcome of Foucault's theoretical work on psychiatry, transforming his criticism into a political struggle. Di Vittorio's stance, albeit otherwise limited to a socio-historical and biographical comparison between Basaglia and Foucault, pinpoints the central idea that when Basaglia refers to a *nodo* between madness and reason, he does not do so in order to describe the history, the 'verità storica', or the conditions of such a relationship. Rather, the socio-historical reflection is the basis from which Basaglia advances possible strategies to counteract the effects of such a historical truth, i.e. that madness is somehow grafted onto the world of reason.

In this chapter, I focus on Basaglia's writings that belong to the phases of institutional negation and deinstitutionalisation proper, from 1964's 'La distruzione dell'ospedale psichiatrico' to his 1980 commentary on Law 180. Biographically, these phases correspond to Basaglia's work in three different psychiatric hospitals: Gorizia (1961–69), Colorno (1969–71) and Trieste (1971–79), with the addition of the short period before his death in 1980, during which Basaglia was appointed director of psychiatric health care services in the region of Lazio and travelled to Brazil. A number of central ideas guided his work in the three above-mentioned asylums. These will be the focus of this chapter, while the reader is referred to Donnelly's work (1994) and to Lovell and Scheper-Hughes's edited volume for a more detailed recounting of the historical and political implications of Basaglia's actions, and to Colucci and Di Vittorio's (2001) and Zanetti and Parmegiani's (2007) biographies for more detailed historical and biographical accounts.

After introducing the main transformations that Basaglia and his team carried out in the asylum at Gorizia, I discuss why he regarded them as insufficient to properly reform biological and institutional psychiatric health care and how the psychiatrist must take advantage of the inpatient's aggressiveness for this purpose. In connection with this, Basaglia's famous motto 'mettere tra parentesi la malattia mentale' is introduced, discussing how it forms a continuum with his criticism of the medical nature of psychiatry and the power that psychiatrists derive from being regarded as physicians. In this criticism and in Basaglia's work of reform in general, two central notions emerge: that of contradiction and that of utopia. Both are, to different extents, involved in the process of overcoming institutional and disciplinary psychiatry. In this process, the psychiatrist plays the part of an *engagé* intellectual, a comparison that Basaglia explicitly outlined. I conclude the chapter with an analysis of the law that sanctioned the 'destruction of the psychiatric hospital', Law 180/1978 and the comments that it engendered.

Reforming the Institution

Basaglia first began working in an asylum in the climate of crisis and protest that I discussed in the previous chapter. In Italy the situation was all the more serious as psychiatric health care was still regulated by a law dating back to 1904, the *Legge 14 Febbraio 1904, n.36*, which defined the *disposizioni sui manicomi e gli internati*. Law 36 associated mental illness with social dangerousness and public scandal, entrusting asylums with the custody and containment of these. The 1904 Italian psychiatric law was consistent with Foucault's portrayal of a science whose main function is that of containing anti-social behaviour, albeit concealing containment in the guise of a necessary medical intervention. To put it in Basaglia's words (1964a: 17), Law 36/1904 was 'una legge antica, ancora incerta fra l'assistenza e la sicurezza, la pietà e la paura'. The very text of the law sanctioned this ambiguous position: 'debbono essere *custodite* e *curate* nei manicomi le persone affette [...] da alienazione mentale' (*art*. 1, added emphases). Asylums were meant to guard 'mental aliens' but also to cure them.

In such conditions it was all the more difficult to put into practice a therapeutic approach such as the one Basaglia advocated in his early works: to treat the patient as a subject and an individual regardless of the psychiatric diagnosis, respecting the distance entailed in an 'authentic' relationship. The total institution of the asylum served a social purpose, that of containing anti-social behaviour, and was certainly not designed to satisfy the needs of those suffering from a mental disorder. If anything, it was thought to make the management of the inmates easier: locked wards, cage-beds and other means of physical restraint (e.g. handcuffs, straitjackets, etc.), shock therapies used to stun the inmate, psychosurgery to make the stunning permanent. The asylum served society by containing deviants, it served the staff by making this task easier, but it did not do much for the inpatient, who was, to all effects and purposes, an inmate of the total institution. In this situation, it is not difficult to understand that a stay in the asylum (often a lifelong internment) had devastating effects on the psychiatric patient. Following the example of others such as Barton (1959) and Wing (1962), Basaglia defined the effects of 'istituzionalizzazione' as 'il complesso di "danni" derivati da un lungo soggiorno coatto quale quello nell'ospedale psichiatrico, quando l'istituto si basi su principi di autoritarismo e di coercizione' (Basaglia, 1965b: 259). According to Basaglia, the effects of institutionalisation are not dissimilar from the symptoms of many mental illnesses. The institution, allegedly built to cure mental illness, actually causes or at least strengthens it; the asylum is a medical yet also paradoxically pathogenic institution:

> l'istituzionalizzazione [è] un comportamento legato al processo di 'rimpicciolimento' dell'io cui il malato mentale è sottoposto dal momento del suo ingresso nell'asilo. Tale processo si sovrapporrebbe, in soggetti già psichicamente fragili, all'iniziale malattia mentale così da costituirne un complesso sindromico che spesso può venir confuso coi sintomi della malattia stessa: inibizioni, apatia, perdita di iniziativa, di interessi, ecc. (Basaglia, 1965b: 259)

The first and most urgent step to starting the transformation of this clearly unacceptable situation was, for Basaglia, to transform the institution itself from the inside. With this in mind, Basaglia discontinued the use of the white coat, a first attempt at symbolically reducing the distance between doctor and patient. Just like uniforms, white coats

> not only allow outsiders to identify individuals as members of the organization but also enabl[e] insiders to interpret their rank, duties, and privileges [...] a basic relation of power, or who controls whom, is conveyed through organizational use of uniforms. (Kaiser, 1990: 362)

Blumhagen (1979), among others, has studied the evolution of the white coat as the respected symbol of medicine. Introduced in 1889 as a means of avoiding cross-contamination it soon became a symbol of purity and moral integrity on the one hand, while on the other, it conferred on physicians and medicine the authority of science. More recently, Wear has studied the hidden implications of the white coat and pointed out that

> wearing the white coat, the occupational clothing of a prestigious group with substantial power over human lives, may actually promote unselfconsciousness. (Wear, 1998: 736)

In short, 'doctors may become the coat' (Wear, 1998: 736). In abandoning it, psychiatrists are thus renouncing not only the uniform that distances them from patients but also the symbol of knowledge and power that the status of physician gives them.

The second step, which Basaglia enforced in Gorizia, was to abolish all forms of physical restraint (such as straitjackets) and physical barriers (such as fencing and iron grilles). Although this initially raised concerns with regard to staff security, the apprehension soon proved unfounded, also thanks in part to the newly introduced antipsychotic drugs (Basaglia, 1964a: 22). Contextually, Basaglia also called for a direct involvement between staff and inmates: the role of the nurses was no longer to keep the inpatients docile and the role of the psychiatrist was no longer to quickly pass through the wards once a day. In Ongaro Basaglia's words (1987: xv), 'doctors could not stay on the wards for a few minutes [and] nurses could no longer calmly play cards'. As all staff were charged with new responsibilities and duties, they did not always appreciate Basaglia's work. Even the pioneer of the therapeutic community, the English psychiatrist Maxwell

Jones, acknowledged similar problems. In his words, 'to have a senior staff member accept discussion and criticism [...] by other staff members, or even patients, is difficult' (Jones, 1968: XX). In this respect, Basaglia (1968c: 475) maintained that

> bisogna che noi stessi – gli appaltatori del potere e della violenza – prendiamo coscienza di essere a nostra volta esclusi, nel momento stesso in cui siamo oggettivati nel nostro ruolo di escludenti.

Those who worked in a psychiatric institution – physicians, nurses, etc. – were often unaware that they themselves were alienated by adopting the role they played: they were part of a logic of suppression and containment of anti-social behaviour, and their medical knowledge was little more than a decoy for this logic.

> [L']*establishment* [...] vuole che gli garantiamo di essere in grado di espletare – tecnicamente – il nostro compito, senza scosse né deviazioni dalla norma: vuole cioè che garantiamo il nostro appoggio e la nostra tecnica a sua difesa e tutela. Nell'accettazione del nostro mandato sociale, noi garantiamo dunque un atto terapeutico che non è che un atto di violenza verso l'escluso, che ci viene affidato perché ne controlliamo tecnicamente le reazioni nei confronti dell'escludente. (Basaglia, 1968c: 475)

In order to reverse the relationship between staff and inpatients, Basaglia adopted a modified version of the 'therapeutic community', inspired by Maxwell Jones's work in Dingleton, Scotland. Basaglia's *assemblee* drew on Maxwell Jones's approach but, as Lovell and Scheper-Hughes (1987: 14) note, were

> not to be confused with the general meetings that were part of the British and American therapeutic community models. The Italian *assemblea* was a stage for confrontation, for expression by people who had been silent for years.

Each day, inmates, nurses and psychiatrists met in a common assembly to discuss outcomes, issues, developments, proposals and also everyday aspects of life inside the asylum. During these meetings, the inmates were allowed to speak, to express their needs and to negotiate with the members of staff for the first time. Whereas in Britain the therapeutic community was generally regarded as a 'technique for collective management', in Gorizia it represented a 'powerful means of unleashing new and dynamic relationships' (Donnelly, 1992: 45).[1] In other words, the therapeutic community aimed at reaching a state of equality, risky as this might have seemed:

> Se finora il malato mentale ha pagato con la segregazione per l'incolumità della società, sta in noi ora pagare il rischio della sua libertà. (Basaglia, 1965c: 291)

Reaching a state of equality meant acknowledging the patients' needs above the needs of the members of staff or the institutional and social requirements, even if this could engender anti-social behaviour.

Besides importing and modifying the therapeutic community, Basaglia applied several other reforms. He made most of the wards of the asylum open, created a day hospital and, at a later stage and especially in Trieste, a 'propaggine dei servizi urbani all'interno dell'ospedale' (Basaglia, 1968f: 24), such as a barber's, a cinema and a social club. These services were aimed at facilitating a merger between cities and asylums, which were usually built in the periphery precisely to separate the 'sane' from the 'insane'. As Pitrelli (2004: 94) remarked, this was a 'restituzione reciproca fra città e ospedale psichiatrico di spazi e di persone'.

Nevertheless, according to Basaglia, a proper reform of psychiatric health care could not be limited to transforming the institution. Undoubtedly, this internal reform 'ha avuto ed ha il compito di demistificare l'ideologia del manicomio' (Basaglia, 1968b: 6). Even so, Basaglia (1968b: 5) acknowledged that 'le nuove contraddizioni che si evidenziano non possono che venire coperte e soffocate attraverso l'ideologia comunitaria che le spiega, le scioglie e le risolve'. The community approach, incarnated in the therapeutic community, the abolishment of physical restraint and in the open wards policy, becomes an abstract ideology comparable with the old institutional closed-door psychiatry when it ceases to be an act of protest and is just adopted as a new and more effective technique for the treatment of mental illness.

---

1   To date, the most comprehensive account of such *assemblee* can be found in the collection of minutes Giovanna Gallio edited for the journal *aut aut* (Gallio, 2009b).

The Risks of Internal Reform

As his paper 'La distruzione dell'ospedale psichiatrico' shows, as early as 1964, Basaglia (1964a: 24) was aware that reforming the institution ran the risk of creating a 'gabbia d'oro'. This 'golden cage' would give rise to a 'stato di soggezione ancora più alienante, perché frammisto a sentimenti di dedizione e riconoscenza che legano [il paziente] al medico' (Basaglia, 1964a: 24). Humanising the conduct of psychiatric health care does not necessarily imply undermining psychiatric power. A psychiatry based on the therapeutic community creates a technical answer to the problem of mental illness, that is, a new and more effective therapy, which 'guarisce di più come OMO lava più bianco'[2] (Basaglia, 1968c: 503). This approach may actually render psychiatry more 'humane' and may also be more effective as far as therapy is concerned. However, even if it does not directly address the need to control deviance, it still fulfils that need. A humanised psychiatric hospital serves the same social purpose as the traditional asylum and can be equally institutionalising. In some respects, this 'istituzionalizzazione molle' (Basaglia, 1964a: 25) would even reinforce psychiatric power, as it would create docile and grateful inmates who would regard the physician as a source of freedom and recovery. In such an 'istituzione della tolleranza' (Basaglia, 1968d: 80) – which is nothing more than the 'faccia adialettica dell'istituzione violenta' (Basaglia, 1969b: 188) – the patient would see healing only as a gift from the psychiatrist and not as a personal conquest, in that he would tend to become 'il perfetto ricoverato':

> ammansito, docile al volere degli infermieri e del medico, quello che si lascia vestire senza reagire, che si lascia pulire, imboccare, che si offre per essere riassettato come si riassetta la sua stanza il mattino; il malato che non complica le cose con reazioni personali, ma si adegua supinamente all'autorità che lo tutela. È il ricoverato di cui si dice – con soddisfazione – che si è ben adattato all'ambiente, che collabora con l'infermiere e con il medico, che si comporta bene con gli altri e non crea complicazioni né opposizioni. (Basaglia, 1965c: 287)

---

2 The ubiquitous detergent 'OMO' used the slogan 'OMO washes whiter' throughout the 1950s and early 1960s in many western countries.

Against the risk of producing docile inpatients, woven into the texture of the institution much like Foucault's docile bodies, Basaglia argued for taking advantage of their aggressiveness. If an equal relationship can be established without a regression into an 'istituzionalizzazione molle', he says, 'l'unico punto su cui sembra di poter far leva è l'aggressività individuale' (Basaglia, 1964a: 25), a conclusion that seemingly draws Basaglia dangerously near to Fanon's argument for 'absolute violence' in the total revolution. Although Fanon had indeed been a source of influence for Basaglia, taking advantage of the inpatient's individual aggressiveness does not involve any violence at all. It does, however, entail a revolutionary stance. The aim of the psychiatrist inside the institution should be 'risvegliare [nel paziente] un sentimento di opposizione al potere che lo ha finora determinato ed istituzionalizzato' (Basaglia, 1965c: 290). Taking advantage of the inpatient's aggressiveness means to stir up the discontent patients manifest towards any aspect of their lives in the asylum rather than restraining or sedating it as if it were yet another symptom of their mental illness. Instead of praising the adapted and cooperative inpatient, the aim is to return to patients the freedom to dissent, give voice to their opinions and oppose the status quo, the basic rights that they had lost upon admission to the asylum. It is not by chance that, in Gorizia, Basaglia introduced the therapeutic community by beginning with the 'reparto agitati', the 'violent' psychiatric ward.

Taking advantage of the patients' aggressiveness was therefore meant to overcome the inpatients' exclusion: let their needs emerge, channel their dissent against the institution of psychiatry, and establish a relationship of reciprocal tension with the members of staff. However, this strategy must not be thought of as a radical form of rehabilitation. If the old-fashioned, excluding and violent psychiatric 'therapy', founded on institutionalisation, physical restraint and submission, is unacceptable, so too is finding a better, more humane and more efficient way of dealing with mental illness – 'come OMO lava più bianco'. In other words, reforming psychiatry does not mean privileging integration over exclusion. Deinstitutionalisation is problematic insofar as it unveils an uncomfortable truth: in a capitalist society integration is not the alternative to exclusion, because both, ultimately, answer to a dominant social logic, that the abnormal has either to be excluded or normalised.

Both the psychiatrist and the inpatient need, therefore, to refuse 'anche l'ultima, mistificata soluzione che viene [loro] proposta: quella dell'integrazione' (Basaglia, 1967c: 419). Integration is a myth not only because it reintroduces sick people into a society that is structurally built on their exclusion as deviants but also because 'la nostra società – pur delegando i tecnici a riabilitarli – non sa che farsene dei malati recuperati' (Basaglia, 1968b: 8). Therefore, the process of adaptation to the dominant norm, whose ultimate aim, as I will discuss at length later, is to assign an active role to the patient in the productive cycle, is not expected to be successful. This makes of integration an ideological chimaera, constructed with the purpose of humanising psychiatric assistance without changing its social mandate.

Basaglia was very sceptical of 'social' psychiatry, the precise aim of which was to reintegrate the sick person into mainstream society. Also, he distrusted human sciences *tout court*, when they proposed an alternative to institutional psychiatry without undermining its presuppositions. 'Il nuovo psichiatra sociale, lo psicoterapeuta, l'assistente sociale, lo psicologo di fabbrica, il sociologo industriale' (Basaglia, 1968c: 474) cannot reform psychiatric assistance insofar as they do not question their own social role. The reason for this is that social psychiatry and the human sciences lack 'l'analisi di quanto costituisce e fonda il sociale cui si riferisc[ono]' (Basaglia, 1970b: 108). It is impossible to radically reform psychiatry if there is no analysis of the social structure which created, motivated and accounted for it as an instrument of control. Without a social and political analysis these social and health care workers are 'i nuovi amministratori della violenza del potere' (Basaglia, 1968c: 474). Their action, 'apparentemente riparatrice e non violenta' (Basaglia, 1968c: 474), is merely another technique that perpetuates institutional power.

Eventually, the years spent working in the asylum also led Basaglia to a critical rethinking of his previous stance, to the point that he put even phenomenological psychiatry under close scrutiny. In his opinion, phenomenological and existentialist approaches to psychiatry had not been able to overcome the objectification of the patient. As he said in 'Le istituzioni della violenza',

> il potere eversivo di questi metodi di approccio si mantiene all'interno di una struttura psicopatologica dove, anziché mettere in discussione l'oggettivazione che viene fatta del malato, si continuano ad analizzare i vari modi di oggettualità. (Basaglia, 1968c: 477)

The phenomenological approach to psychiatry itself is still very far from the 'realtà cui avrebbe dovuto riferirsi' (Basaglia, 1970a: 137). Phenomenological psychiatry still dictates a framework that foregrounds the actual experience of madness and can be regarded as an *a priori* approach to the patient.

Yet it is no easy task to overcome such an approach in the asylum and to begin analysing the social structures that made of psychiatry – biological, institutional or even social – such a discriminating, stigmatising and, ultimately, non-medical endeavour. In the psychiatric hospital, as Goffman (2007: 306) observes:

> whatever the patient's social circumstances, whatever the particular character of his 'disorder', he can [...] be treated as someone whose problem can be approached, if not dealt with, by applying a single technical-psychiatric view.

If the patient's symptoms are only interpreted as the signs of an illness, the patient's needs will be met only from a technical-psychiatric point of view. As a matter of fact, Basaglia (1975b: 357) did not intend to assert that mental illness does not exist,

> ma che noi produciamo una sintomatologia [...] a seconda del modo col quale pensiamo di gestire [la malattia], perché la malattia si costruisce e si esprime sempre a immagine delle misure che si adottano per affrontarla.

The theoretical framework adopted when assessing behaviour shapes behaviour itself. This rules out the possibility that what psychiatry reads as a symptom could be instead an act of disagreement, rebellion or even subjective expression against the impositions of society. Hence, the inmate is somehow denied freedom of expression because 'ogni atto di contestazione alla realtà che vive [è] solo sintomo di malattia' (Basaglia, 1967c: 417). Once the psychiatrist diagnoses a mental illness, the institution completely relieves patients of any responsibility, as it interprets every single action of theirs as a mere symptom.

If patients' often violent protests against physical restraint, their insubordination or even their unsatisfied needs are seen as symptoms of an illness, to the point that recovery is equated to docile subordination, psychiatric intervention is still regulated by what Basaglia called a 'metafisica dogmatica'. Patients might well have been interned in the asylum mainly because of anti-social behaviour, yet because they *are* in the asylum, the staff will automatically, *a priori*, treat them as sick. The entirety of their behaviour will be understood under the label of mental illness, all of the staff's actions towards patients will be labelled 'therapeutic intervention' and any changes in the patients' lives will be read in the dichotomy regression/recovery. In this narrow context, there is no space of an analysis of the social structures that might have forced patients into certain anti-social behaviours in the first place, or the staff into the positions of power they occupy, for that matter. For these reasons, Basaglia believed that, first and foremost mental illness had to be 'put in brackets'.

'Bracketing' Mental Illness

According to Basaglia (1968d: 81), we do not know much about madness. The organic hypotheses on mental illness and its possible medical treatments 'sono rimaste ipotesi non verificate'. Yet as he (1975b: 358) puts it, 'cancro e malattia mentale esistono come fatti concreti' and, in his opinion, this is indisputable. Basaglia never denied the existence of mental illness or its possible biological roots: a mental illness is a 'contraddizione che si verifica in un contesto sociale'. For this reason, it is not only a social product but 'una interazione tra tutti i livelli di cui noi siamo composti: biologico, sociale, psicologico' (Basaglia, 2000: 99). However, in this multifaceted dimension, the psychiatrist can move only from one premise:

> ciò che sappiamo è che abbiamo a che fare con dei malati e che siamo costantemente tentati di coprire la contraddizione che essi rappresentano ai nostri occhi con un'ideologia, per cercarne la soluzione (Basaglia, 1968d: 80).

The only way to avoid concealing the contradiction that the sick person represents is to 'mettere tra parentesi la malattia mentale' (Basaglia, 1966b: 44); that is to say, to omit 'ogni definizione nosografica' or to disregard 'la malattia come fatto reale' (Basaglia, 1969a: 35–36). As Colucci and Di Vittorio (2001: 27*ff*) have observed, Basaglia's 'bracketing' of mental illness resembles Husserl's *epoché*. Briefly, in his *Ideas: General Introduction to Pure Phenomenology* (Husserl, 1931), Husserl defined *epoché* as the suspension of judgement concerning the true nature of reality. Only through such a suspension is it possible to carry out a phenomenological investigation whose aims are not governed by preconceptions and prejudices. Yet, as opposed to Husserl's *epoché*, Basaglia's 'bracketing' of mental illness does not involve reality as such (Basaglia, 1981a: xxii). The psychiatrist has to 'bracket' the assumptions on mental illness, which basically derive from the twofold perspective that Foucault also highlights and that underpins even the formulation of Law 36/1904: the medical perspective (i.e. madness is an illness) and the social/moral (i.e. madness amounts to danger and scandal). More recently, Raymond McCall has returned to the importance of *epoché* in psychiatry. McCall distinguishes three different forms of *epoché*: the 'bracketing' of all the non-psychological elements of his investigation (such as behaviour, physical reality, etc.); the so-called transcendental reduction, which aims at referring the subject only to his self-consciousness; and finally phenomenological reduction *stricto sensu*, which means 'to overcome the illusions of perfect objectivity' (McCall, 1983: 56–59). This phenomenological reduction grants the psychiatrist several insights.

First of all, biological and institutional psychiatry considered the patient through the supposedly objective lens of medicine. In *Asylums*, Goffman (2007: 306) had already noted that psychiatry reduced all the possible approaches to the patient to a technical-psychiatric perspective. From this point of view, the psychiatrist cannot distinguish between behaviour on the part of patients which is a direct consequence and manifestation of their illness, in other words, an actual symptom of it, and behaviour which is assumed to be a symptom for the sole purpose of classifying patients' anti-social or abnormal behaviour. This was precisely Basaglia's concern. 'Bracketing' mental illness would mean skipping the need to diagnose a patient's behaviour within the set boundaries of a mental illness, thus allegedly making it possible to prioritise the intersubjective relationship with the patient over the medical study of the illness.

Secondly, 'bracketing' allowed the psychiatrist to 'individuare quale parte avesse giocato nel processo di distruzione del malato la malattia e quale l'istituzione' (Basaglia, 1981b: xxii). In other words, 'bracketing' mental illness enabled the psychiatrist to distinguish between the negative effects of institutionalisation and the suffering that pre-existed institutionalisation. In doing so, 'bracketing' revealed that inmates might be expressing certain unsatisfied needs through their behaviour, which was classed as a symptom of the mental illness. In fact, the aim of institutional psychiatry had been 'la tutela dell'ordine pubblico' and certainly not a 'risposta al bisogno espresso dalla malattia' (Basaglia, 1975b: 359). 'Bracketing' mental illness made it possible for the psychiatrist to allow the effects that the imposition of social norms had on the sick person to emerge.

From these considerations, it follows that the psychiatrist should act on both the biological and the social aspect of the illness. Biological therapy, though, had been lagging behind during the 1950s and early 1960s, especially in Italy. Before the widespread implementation of anti-psychotic drugs, psychiatric therapies were limited. Administering a 'physical' therapy, such as electroconvulsive therapy, therefore, proved controversial. In spite of the rather successful attempts made by the American Psychiatric Association to standardise psychiatric nosography in the *Diagnostic and Statistic Manual of Mental Disorders* (first edition in 1952, second in 1968), in psychiatry, unlike in other medical specialties, nosography was – and still is – an open matter of debate, consequently undermining the creation of consistent and stable diagnostic criteria. Therapeutic methods were often used without a solid scientific study as to their efficacy, and prognosis was highly uncertain and depended on several non-medical factors, such as the social context, the conditions of life in the asylum, etc. On the other hand, the alternatives to institutionalisation were available only to those who could afford a private clinic (it must be borne in mind that the asylum was financed by the provinces or the regions, in accordance with art. 1 of Law 36/1904). Hence, the decision as to who was to be confined in an asylum and who was to be treated in a clinic ultimately depended on their economic condition.

For these reasons, the psychiatrist, as a physician, could not do much that targeted the organic aspect of mental illness. However, according to Basaglia, psychiatrists could be very effective if they worked on a social and political level, without entailing an explicit recourse to social psychiatry. That is to say, 'mettere tra parentesi la malattia mentale' disclosed the social aspect of mental illness, with all its implications and consequences: the stigmatising effects of institutionalisation on the patient, the social structures that support psychiatry as a means of social control, the pathogenetic effects of the imposition of social norms, etc. In Basaglia's words (1969a: 36), 'ciò che viene affrontato e discusso, attraverso la messa tra parentesi della malattia, è il suo aspetto sociale'. In other words, psychiatrists discovered that patients suffered first and foremost from a lack of correspondence between their individual needs and social norms rather than exclusively from an illness.

Hence, bracketing mental illness calls into question the problem of normativity in society as such. In other words, it enables an analysis of the basis on which society, especially a capitalist society, fabricates norms. According to Basaglia, in the contemporary capitalist system the most important of norms concerns productivity: the normal individual is the one who is productive, whereas deviants are those who are unproductive. As early as the 1968 article 'La comunità terapeutica e le istituzioni psichiatriche', Basaglia insisted that institutional psychiatry considers the sick person as 'un elemento di disturbo, da escludere'. The cause for this exclusion is precisely 'il fatto [...] di essere usciti dal processo produttivo' (Basaglia, 1968b: 7). Here his thought overlaps with Foucault's: the distinction between normal and abnormal in a capitalist society is the criterion of productivity: the normal, productive, dominant group of individuals (the middle class, the bourgeoisie) entrusts psychiatry with the control of unproductive individuals, on the grounds of their being 'the most immediate threat' to the bourgeois order (Foucault, 2006a: 379).

Revealing this distinction further problematises the very assumptions that underpin the capitalist system. According to Basaglia, there is a certain confusion between social norms and economic logic at the heart of the discrimination between normal and abnormal. In the entry on the theme of 'Follia/Delirio' in the Einaudi Encyclopaedia, Basaglia (1979a: 429) claims that 'il corpo economico è contrabbandato come un corpo sociale'. While the needs of people should shape the social body, this is clearly not the case in a capitalist society, where the institutions that support the economic body also shape the social one. As a consequence, the capitalist social body, with its norms, institutions and prejudices, is the result of an economic logic based on profit. Therefore, it cannot respond to the actual needs of people. Eventually, this situation produces individuals who are alienated by the economic logic and are 'implicitamente subordinat[i] alle esigenze della logica che l[i] determina' (Basaglia, 1979a: 429).

Basaglia supports his argument with a statistical study that he conducted along with his team in the asylums at Trieste and Volterra. The data shows that the number of hospitalisations and discharges followed the general course of economy; that is to say, higher hospitalisation rates corresponded to periods of economic recession and higher rates of discharges to periods of economic development. It seems as though:

> a seconda dei diversi momenti di sviluppo o di recessione e di crisi, si assiste al contemporaneo allargamento o restringimento dei limiti di norma e, quindi, al dilatarsi o restringersi della tolleranza nei confronti dei comportamenti anormali. (Basaglia, 1976: 386)[3]

In a period of economic recession individuals are required to be more productive; as the social body cannot provide for those who are unproductive, the norm 'shrinks', and the exclusion of deviants increases. Conversely, in periods of economic growth, the social body can look after unproductive individuals; in this case, the norm 'expands', allowing a more generous tolerance of deviants.

The most important outcome of the 'bracketing' of mental illness is precisely the revelation of the economic bias underlying psychiatry. This bias explains, for instance, why the majority of inmates in an asylum were the impoverished and the destitute, who lacked the economic means to survive in a capitalist society and needed to be somehow contained by it.

---

3   The relevant data can be found in Basaglia, 1976: 387.

For this reason, the process of 'bracketing' mental illness calls into question the social structures that support institutional psychiatry and its discriminatory methods. However, bracketing mental illness also entails criticising those alternative psychiatric treatments that were aimed at reforming institutional psychiatry, such as social psychiatry and *Daseinsanalyse* itself. These alternatives, while effectively humanising psychiatry, could not change the social structures that grounded institutional psychiatry. Hence, they would only replace it with a treatment serving the same purpose of containing unproductive individuals.

All things considered, we could say that this comes down to the fact that psychiatry is a branch of medicine that specialises in the treatment of mental illness: if not biological psychiatrists then someone else must be eventually entrusted with tackling madness. The problem, as I have extensively discussed so far, is not how effectively one deals with madness, but why all the modes of dealing with madness entail it being classed as a disease and dealt with as far as possible from 'sane' society. We have seen that Foucault regards the process that made of psychiatry a medical science nothing short of a 'dense mystery'. What I will focus on in the next section is a similar conundrum that Basaglia unearths in his work: the fact that psychiatry is taken to belong among the medical specialisms contributes to its being entrusted with the social mandate of containing deviance. However, having to contain deviance, psychiatry is unable to actually help and heal the mental patient, although this is the reason why psychiatry was regarded as a medical specialism in the first place.

Psychiatry and Medicine

Being regarded as a medical specialism, psychiatry is supposed to be an unbiased, objective and specialised application of medicine to mental disorders; that is to say, it should not be hindered by moral, social or economic considerations. However, especially after the great wave of 'anti-psychiatry' in the 1960s, this could hardly be upheld. Interestingly, some scholars went as far as calling into question even the alleged unbiased and scientific nature of medicine itself. One of those scholars was Michel Foucault.

In his 1963 *Naissance de la clinique* (*The Birth of the Clinic*) Foucault, following Canguilhem's work among others, argues that contemporary medicine is based on a certain clinical 'gaze' (*regard*), which treats the dead, anatomical body and its diseased components as the visible objects of a positive science. This objective and supposedly neutral 'gaze' is a concept whose history is entwined with power relations and economic reasons (Foucault, 2008a). With regard to the historical nature of medicine, Sigerist (1932: 35) asserts that 'medicine is closely associated with general culture, that every change in medical thinking is the outcome of the world point of view of the time'. Canguilhem (2007: 103) relies on Sigerist to endorse the idea that a medical concept seems 'to satisfy simultaneously several demands and intellectual postulates of the historical moment of the culture in which it was formulated'. According to these studies, the main issue is not that psychiatry cannot be considered to be a medical science but that medicine itself cannot be unquestionably regarded as an unbiased scientific endeavour. As Canguilhem (2007: 221–22) says, every scientific perspective is 'an abstract point of view' insofar as it expresses 'a choice and hence a neglect'. This choice tends to privilege those objects that allow 'measurement and casual explanation'. The 'need to determine scientifically what is real', i.e. what is measurable, extends also to life, with the so-called sciences of life and especially with medicine. In *The Birth of the Clinic*, Foucault (2008a: xx) advances a possible 'analysis of a type of discourse, that of medical experience', which we are 'accustomed to recognising as the language of a "positive science"'. As Rose (1999: 52) observes, Foucault's analysis reveals 'the political objectives [that] have been specified in the vocabularies and grammars of medicine'. Foucault's analysis thus breaks medicine down into a series of political and social effects. In Rose's words (1999: 55), 'medicine [...] has played a formative role in the *invention of the social*'. More recently, Žižek returns to this point by extending his critique to the sciences in general. According to Žižek (2009: 69), 'science today effectively does compete with religion'. It does so, insofar as science is as ideological as religion, because 'it serves two properly ideological needs, those for hope and those for censorship'. In this way, science first and foremost works as a 'social force, as an ideological institution'. Science has become a universal discourse, an absolute 'point of reference' that is hardly questioned.

According to Basaglia (1968e: 468), these considerations are all the more true in psychiatry. In this discipline, the aura of scientific neutrality eventually 'agisce a sostegno dei valori dominanti'. It does so, insofar as it conceals the true social and economic considerations that ground psychiatry. Arguably, psychiatry, especially as it was practised in Italy before Basaglia, was not a neutral medical science either, in that its dealings with patients by and large had a socioeconomic bias; as Ongaro Basaglia (1987: xvi) observes, 'the discourse about the nonneutrality of science […] found a practical confirmation in the Gorizia experience'. While private and university clinics admitted those patients who could afford the high fees involved, hospitalisation in the public asylum, financed by the provinces, was free of charge. Hence, although institutional psychiatry was also dealing with mental illness, it came to treat only the patients belonging to the lower classes, those who could not afford private facilities. As Basaglia (1975a: 239) observes, 'il manicomio non è l'ospedale per chi soffre di disturbi mentali, ma il luogo di contenimento di certe devianze di comportamento degli appartenenti alla classe subalterna'.

Although Basaglia seems to be suggesting that belonging to a subordinate class is a sufficient precondition to being regarded as potentially dangerous, this issue is not further developed in his writings. However, he does stress how the aura of scientific neutrality and the notion of psychiatry as a specialised medical knowledge contribute to better concealing its ultimate purpose of social control. As he says,

> non è automatico che la classe subalterna, anche la più politicizzata, riconosca nella scienza e nelle ideologie la manipolazione e il controllo di cui è oggetto, e non invece un valore assoluto, che accetta perché al di là della propria possibilità di conoscere e di comprendere. (Basaglia, 1975a: 244)

The medical science of psychiatry enjoys the objectivity and neutrality of other sciences and is a specialised form of knowledge, with technicians specialised in its study and clinical application, i.e. psychiatrists. Inasmuch as they draw their conclusions (diagnoses, prognoses, treatments, etc.) from allegedly scientific, neutral and objective observations, their decisions are not to be challenged except by an equally specialised expertise. Madness is a real, observable and treatable illness only inasmuch as there is an allegedly scientific knowledge that defines it so. Given that this knowledge pertains to a specialised domain, those who have not specialised in psychiatry cannot properly understand mental illness. Psychiatric symptoms as much as physical symptoms are in fact 'inaccessible to the patient without a medical interpretation' (Armstrong, 1995: 19). Only specialised workers can provide such an interpretation. The impossibility for untrained people to understand and call into question psychiatric knowledge conceals all the more, according to Basaglia, the economic and social grounds of psychiatric practice.

The Contradictory Situation of Deinstitutionalisation

In Gorizia, then, Basaglia and his team were in a controversial situation. They were still the representatives of the medical science of psychiatry, although they had got rid of the white coats. They could bracket mental illness, humanise everyday life in the asylum, abolish violent and pathogenetic treatments, take advantage of the patient's aggressiveness to establish a relationship of reciprocal tension between the patient and the psychiatrist, return freedom of expression to the inpatient, and so on. Yet to what end? To keep the sick as inpatients of an 'istituzione della tolleranza' was certainly not an option. Reintegrating the outpatient in the capitalist system was no option either, as the very premise of this system is the exclusion of the unproductive mentally ill person and the maintenance of the bourgeois order. In Basaglia's own words, in Gorizia

[f]inché si resta all'interno del sistema, la nostra situazione non può che continuare ad essere contraddittoria: l'istituzione è contemporaneamente negata e gestita, la malattia è contemporaneamente messa fra parentesi e curata, l'atto terapeutico viene contemporaneamente rifiutato e agito. (Basaglia, 1968a: 515)

The first contradictory situation stems from the opposition between curing and 'bracketing' mental illness. As psychiatrists, Basaglia and his team were being asked to cure mental illness; but as reformers of psychiatry, they were trying to disregard psychiatric 'labels', from very specific diagnoses to the most general notion of mental illness itself. Still in line with Basaglia's early phenomeno-existentialist influence, this was done in order to achieve a deeper *understanding* of each individual patient considered as a subject instead of delivering a scientific *explanation* of their abnormal behaviour. Such an understanding focuses on the two aspects that were neglected in biological and institutional psychiatry: the subjectivity of the patient and the social aspect of the illness. In Basaglia's opinion, the opposition between curing and 'bracketing' mental illness stems from the fact that we do not know what madness is: 'non so cosa sia la follia. Può essere tutto o niente. È una condizione umana' (Basaglia, 2000: 34). Yet, according to Basaglia, biological psychiatry concealed all possible doubts concerning madness by defining it as a mental illness, that is, a phenomenon that can be explained scientifically. By bracketing mental illness, Basaglia tried to operate without silencing this doubt. If psychiatrists do not know what madness is, then they have to 'bracket' all psychiatric *a priori* assumptions. Instead of acting as therapists who need to cure a disease, psychiatrists must face patients as if they were dealing with 'healthy' human beings, albeit marginalised from society. In doing so, they are confronting individuals, social and political subjects, who have to understand themselves as much as their relationship with society.

The opposition between curing and disregarding mental illness ultimately rests on the opposition between health and illness. We are used to considering health as the normal state of life, so illness is seen as an exception to the norm. This reprises the observation Canguilhem (2007: 138) had already made about twenty years before when he said that 'one could say that continual perfect health is abnormal'. If we take the concept of health in an absolute way, it 'is a normative concept defining an ideal type of organic structure and behaviour' (Canguilhem, 2007: 137); yet he continues, 'the experience of living indeed includes disease' (Canguilhem, 2007: 138). Similarly, Basaglia regards both illness and health as opposite yet fundamental conditions of life. In his own words, 'un buon ordinamento sociale dovrebbe fare in modo che il malato viva la propria esperienza di malato come un'esperienza di vita' (Basaglia, 1975b: 359).

Most importantly, Basaglia was perfectly aware of the contradiction that he himself represented as the director of an asylum. He was managing an institution he was also dismantling: 'la contraddizione fra negazione e gestione dell'istituzione è la prima di cui si deve tener conto' (Basaglia, 1975a: 296). In order not to conceal such a contradictory situation, Basaglia could not privilege the pole of institutional negation. This would have prevented him from acknowledging that even '[la negazione] si inserisce all'interno di un'organizzazione e di una ideologia scientifica la cui logica è nostro compito spezzare' (Basaglia, 1975a: 296). It would also lead eventually to an ideology of negation and recreate the relationship of power that existed before the deinstitutionalisation. It would, in other words, recreate the psychiatrist as a new 'appaltatore della violenza', whose task would be 'mistificare – attraverso il tecnicismo – la violenza, senza tuttavia modificarne la natura' (Basaglia, 1968e: 474).

Any reform risks becoming part of the very system it is trying to reform. This can happen when a subversive idea becomes the dominant one, and also when a revolutionary practice becomes a new technical and codified answer to a controversial problem. In this way, instead of being the result of criticism and constant negotiation with the changing reality it turns into the uncritical and repetitive application of an established procedure. In psychiatry, contradictions must be left unresolved in order to avoid 'la cristallizzazione delle risposte' (Basaglia, 1977: 403) into a medical answer to the social problem that madness represents.

Utopias and the Double Presence of Contradictions

Madness itself, in fact, raises many contradictions. Beginning with 'La distruzione dell'ospedale psichiatrico' (1964), Basaglia focused on the contradictory situation that madness raises between individual needs and social norms as well as between subjects who want to be recognised as such and a science that considers them as objects. Encompassing both definitions, Basaglia (2000: 99) claimed that madness as an illness is a contradiction 'del nostro corpo, e dicendo corpo, dico corpo organico e sociale'.

For these reasons, it is of the utmost importance for the psychiatrist to live 'dialetticamente le contraddizioni del reale' (Basaglia, 1964b: 399). To face 'dialectically' both mental illness as a contradiction and the issues thereby raised means that psychiatrists must not silence this contradiction by the explanations of a predetermined ideology. At least in the context of the psychiatric hospital undergoing the process of reform, madness must be considered as a contradiction that cannot be solved and that members of staff must face on a daily basis by dialectically negotiating the possible solutions of each single issue it raises. Biological psychiatry tended to base diagnosis and therapy on *a priori* categories, relating all problematic behaviour by the patient to the standard symptoms of the illness, rather than facing them in their uniqueness.

It follows from this that the concept of contradiction also plays a specific political role in the work of deinstitutionalisation as such. According to Basaglia (1980: 481–82), contradictions were elements in his political strategy, because

> evidenziare le contraddizioni significa creare l'apertura di una spaccatura. [...] Nel tempo che intercorre tra l'esplosione della contraddizione e la sua copertura (perché non può avvenire che questo), si determina un'occasione di presa di coscienza da parte dell'opinione pubblica.

On the one hand, Basaglia suggests that contradictions should be kept unresolved through a continuous negotiation; in such a way, one could deal with the uniqueness of each single individual. On the other hand, when kept unresolved, contradictions generate further dialectical processes, which can go as far as undermining power. This is possible insofar as a contradiction amounts to a double presence. The first is 'la presenza del relativo (quindi del polo concreto del reale, del possibile) all'interno di un discorso che rischia di assolutizzarsi' (Basaglia, 1970b: 124). Possibly, Basaglia is here suggesting that what he refers to as 'real' transcends the mere level of perceived reality. Arguably, the 'real' amounts to the presence of what is relative, local and subjective in the general perception of reality. According to Basaglia, what we perceive as reality is only a product of ideologies: definitions, norms, codifications are 'messi in atto dalla classe dominante per costruire la realtà secondo i propri bisogni' (Basaglia, 1975a: 254). Individual needs and the contradictions to which they give rise are silenced by these ideologies. This is the reason why Basaglia regards them as being the 'real'. The 'concrete pole of the real' is the resistance to the creation of ideologies; that is to say, absolute and abstract representations of reality, aimed at silencing social contradictions, the 'obscene' byproduct of society. As one would expect, this local resistance runs the risk of being turned into a replacement for ideologies and thus of becoming itself a new ideology. Basaglia was concerned that this might happen with the work of deinstitutionalisation, which could have created a new and more effective psychiatric technique to be used uncritically for the same social and political purposes as institutional psychiatry.

Nonetheless, a local resistance not only runs the risk of becoming an ideology: it also runs the risk of remaining a mere local endeavour that does not call into question the general ideology which it was resisting. For instance, Basaglia's work was initially aimed at reforming institutional psychiatry. Yet it risked remaining a local resistance, centred in the Gorizia and Trieste asylums, unable to reach the social structures that *produced* asylums.

A contradiction therefore also amounts to a second kind of presence. It is also 'la presenza dell'assoluto (l'impossibile, ciò che si vuole essere) all'interno di un discorso relativo che porta in sé la propria morte' (Basaglia, 1970b: 124). This 'absolute' would not be ideological insofar as it would not entail norms. It would not impose an abstract representation of society to silence its obscene side. When Basaglia refers to this 'absolute', he is referring to the presence of a utopian aim. The utopian aim should guide local resistance and prevent it from remaining a mere local endeavour with no chance of having an effect on society as a whole. A social contradiction is an opportunity to make people aware of the social injustice that is the byproduct of society itself. This is possible because a social contradiction is the presence of a local resistance to the 'absolutising' power of ideologies and, at the same time, it is also the presence of the utopian aims that guide this local resistance.

In the wake of these considerations, Basaglia (1975a: 254) put forward the idea that reality should be regarded as something that is 'praticamente vero'. Reality should not be regarded as something given and static. It should be regarded as a dynamic entity which is shaped by the actual needs of the people. On the other hand, utopia should be regarded as an 'elemento prefigurante' (Basaglia, 1975a: 254) of this reality. Utopias are 'una ricerca costante sul piano dei bisogni, delle risposte più adeguate alla costruzione di una vita possibile per tutti gli uomini' (Basaglia, 1975a: 254). Reality should be constantly shaped and reshaped, according to this continuous search based on the needs of human beings. If reality is to be regarded as an unstable condition, then utopia is the element that prevents reality from becoming static.

Basaglia's notion of utopia is in stark contrast to all previous understandings of the term in the context of psychiatry. As Lovell and Scheper-Hughes (1987: 1) aptly observe, 'the history of psychiatry is replete with the myth making that perpetuates [...] utopian visions'. Every epistemological break in the history of psychiatry, such as Pinel's freeing the madmen from the chains at *Salpêtrière* hospital, had been moved by a utopian vision. However, this utopian vision was never detached from the need of social control; in Lovell and Scheper-Hughes's words (1987: 3),

> earlier proposals [to reform psychiatry] were utopias in the sense that they generated ideologies, each with a preconceived future that would reinforce and improve upon existing patterns of management and control over excluded groups.

Basaglia's notion of utopia is very distant from this idea, as he urges us to consider utopias as *practical* realities: 'Basaglia's changes were forged out of the specific context in which he worked' (Lovell and Scheper-Hughes,

1987: 3). To this extent, Crossley (1999) used the asylum at Trieste, along with Kingsley Hall, as examples of what he calls 'working utopias'; that is to say 'sites for pedagogic action, experimentation and market places for ideas and social capital [...] sites of embodied practice' (Crossley, 1999: 826), where revolutionary social movements can epitomise the success of their pioneering and reforming reach.

How can such a notion of utopia guide the reforming psychiatric practice in the contradictory situation that Basaglia described? The only possible subversive, albeit necessarily temporary, action that could undermine, from within the institution, the social mandate of psychiatry and limit the power psychiatrists exert on behalf of the dominant class, was 'un'azione che tendeva a fondarsi su forme precarie di organizzazione, che rifiutava di stabilizzarsi su nuove regole positive' (Basaglia, 1977: 392). Society constantly asks the psychiatrist to produce a newer and better technique for controlling and containing anti-social behaviour, be it a radical lobotomy, a violent Cardiazol convulsive therapy or a humane rehabilitative therapeutic community. The only possible way to avoid abiding by this request is to refuse to give a final answer to the problem that madness represents: refusing diagnoses by bracketing mental illness, refusing the conciliating rehabilitation process by taking advantage of the inpatient's aggressiveness.

However, in doing this, Basaglia can no longer confront only the somewhat limited *milieu* of the asylum: it is pointless to give bargaining powers, freedom of expression and the possibility of dissent and revolt back to the patients if they nevertheless remain locked inside the institution. As Mollica (1985: 31) puts it, 'society had to be brought into collision with the problems it had tried to lock away in the asylum', and it is to this extent that, in Basaglia's (1968e: 468) words, 'la polemica al sistema istituzionale esce dalla sfera psichiatrica, per trasferirsi alle strutture sociali che la sostengono'. It is important to stress outright that this is not meant to be a cure for mental illness, as if Basaglia thought that mental illness was exclusively caused by a pathogenetic society and that stirring the inpatients' rebelliousness would suffice to dispel it. On the contrary, acting on a social level and bringing psychiatric issues to the social and political arena meant keeping unresolved the issues that madness represents. It meant proclaiming that the treatment so far administered to the mentally ill in the asylum was not only unacceptable but also and especially symptomatic of a capitalist society where unproductive deviants could not hinder the productive cycle. What is more, it showed that the fate of the inmate in the asylum incarnates the fate of all the underrepresented social strata, Basaglia's *classe subalterna* – indigents, deviants, disabled, but also women, homosexuals, etc. – in the contemporary capitalist system: either they are excluded from society, ostracised, or else normalised and patronisingly reintegrated in a system where they are required to be the docile subalterns.

To this extent, Basaglia equated the figure of the psychiatrist with that of the intellectual. The alternative, reforming psychiatrists have to refuse their social mandate and the privileges it entails and side with the inmates, to defend them against the abuse of the dominant class. Likewise, it was argued that the intellectual, formerly exploited by the dominant class to exert power, had to take the lower classes' side and aid them in their struggle for emancipation.

Psychiatrists and Intellectuals

During the work of reform, psychiatrists are in a precarious condition. In order to support the inmates, they must abandon their traditional position of power; at the same time, they have to question their own knowledge. In doing so, the psychiatrist transcends the *milieu* of the asylum and engages with wider social and political issues. When psychiatrists question their own power and knowledge in order to support the inmates, they engage with the general issues that intellectuals encounter when they side with a subordinate class. Basaglia focuses on the role of intellectuals especially in his article, 'Crimini di pace' (1975a), and in the preface to the book with the same title, which is a collection of papers and interviews focused on the role of intellectuals as technicians of oppression.[4]

When dealing with the figure of the intellectual, Basaglia relies extensively on Antonio Gramsci's theories. In the twelfth of his *Quaderni del carcere*, Gramsci (1977: 1512) states that while 'tutti gli uomini sono intellettuali [...] non tutti gli uomini hanno, nella società, funzione di intellettuali'. Gramsci distinguishes two types of intellectuals *stricto sensu*, i.e. those who have an intellectual function in society: traditional and organic intellectuals. The former pre-exist the rise to power of a dominant class (as regards the historical period that interests us here, the dominant class is indubitably the bourgeoisie). The first task of a rising class is the 'assimilazione e conquista ideologica' (Gramsci, 1977: 1517) of the traditional intellectual. At the same time, the dominance of the emerging social group is all the stronger if the group is able to create its own 'organic intellectuals'. These form an organic whole with political power, and are created exclusively to facilitate the exertion of power. Both co-opted traditional intellectuals and organic ones are therefore 'commessi del gruppo dominante per l'esercizio delle funzioni subalterne dell'egemonia sociale e del governo politico' (Gramsci, 1977: 1519). Their purpose is to exert power on behalf of the dominant class by enforcing cultural hegemony. Gramsci thus advances that it is now time for the lower classes, the subaltern classes, to train their own 'intellettuali organici', to exert a counter-cultural hegemony against the dominant bourgeoisie.

In line with Gramsci, Basaglia (1975a: 241) asserts that the intellectual has so far played a 'ruolo di funzionario del consenso'. That is to say, he quotes from Gramsci, intellectuals have had 'il compito di assicurare legalmente la disciplina di quei gruppi che non "consentono" né attivamente né passivamente' (Gramsci, 1977: 1519; quoted in Basaglia, 1975a: 239). Intellectuals have disciplined the subordinate classes, workers, the

[4] Among the most notable contributions to this book edited by Basaglia we should mention Michel Foucault's 'La casa della follia', which includes the Italian version of the *Psychiatric Power* course resumé; Robert Castel's 'La contraddizione psichiatrica'; two essays by the anti-psychiatrists Laing and Szasz and one by the sociologist Erving Goffman.

proletariat, the poor and also the mentally ill. These 'funzionari del consenso' have been able to do so by exercising a certain amount of power on behalf of the dominant class but also, and especially, by being the sole administrators of specific – pedagogic, medical, institutional – techniques that ease the enforcement of cultural hegemony. To this extent, Sartre (1975: 232) refers to them as part of a wider group of 'technicians of practical knowledge'. In Basaglia's words (1975a: 239), they are the

> esecutori materiali delle ideologie [...] gli intellettuali di serie C, [...] coloro che affrontano problemi pratico-teorici, traducendo l'astrazione della teoria nella pratica istituzionale.

The lower classes work to realise aims defined by the ruling ones. Intellectuals make this possible through a series of techniques which contribute to the disciplining of 'quei gruppi che non "consentono" né attivamente né passivamente'. Yet intellectuals exercise power on behalf of the dominant class. Just like the lower classes, the actions of intellectuals do not satisfy their own requirements, in that they are not allowed to express their own needs, because they have to conform to those of the dominant class. In the clear-cut dichotomy between ruling and lower classes, intellectuals play the role of intermediaries. They endorse the claims of dominant ideologies, reinforcing the justifications for exploiting the lower classes and administering techniques to exclude them from ruling positions. Needless to say such a stance is indebted to Marx's reflection. According to him, intellectuals, or ideologists, serve the ruling class inasmuch as they produce ideologies capable of masking the alienating character of labour. In *The German Ideology*, Marx and Engels (1970: 64) point out that 'the class which has the means of material production at its disposal, has control at the same time over the means of mental production, so that thereby, generally speaking, the ideas of those who lack the means of mental production are subject to it'. Having access to the means of 'mental production', the members of the ruling class can impose their needs on the masses of workers: they create ideologies that justify and endorse the existing social arrangements.

In Basaglia's opinion, these considerations can be seamlessly applied to psychiatry. Psychiatrists in general, but especially those working in an asylum, are 'funzionari del consenso' inasmuch as they are entrusted with the identification and custody of social deviants. These 'deviants' are merely those who do not comply with the requirements of the dominant ideology, i.e. those who do not 'consent' (Basaglia, 1975a: 239). Psychiatrists also fit into the category of 'technicians of a practical knowledge'. Institutional psychiatry understood as a 'risposta tecnica a una domanda economica' allows psychiatrists to translate the nosographic knowledge into an alleged therapeutic practice. Yet, although this practice implies a certain amount of power, institutional psychiatrists exercise it only on behalf of the dominant class. They can impose a diagnosis on patients, enforce their hospitalisation and regulate all of their life in the 'total institution' of the asylum. Even so, they cannot modify the essential purpose of their actions: that is, marginalising an individual who is considered deviant.

The role of intellectuals and the extent of their engagement with political and social issues was one of the central topics of debate in the wave of protest in the late 1960s. In this context, it suffices to mention the relationship between Basaglia's conception of the intellectual and Foucault's. Foucault distinguishes two types of intellectuals: the universal and the specific intellectual. Although this distinction is made apparent throughout his late work especially, Foucault defines it very clearly in the 1976 interview 'Truth and Power'. On the one hand, the 'universal intellectual [...] acknowledged the right of speaking in the capacity of master of truth and justice'. That is to say, he considered himself or was considered as 'the spokesman of the universal' (Foucault, 1986: 67), in whose speech 'the tone of prophecy and promised pleasure neatly mesh' (Dreyfus and Rabinow, 1982: 130). Basaglia uses Gramsci's definition of 'funzionario del consenso' for the figure that Foucault refers to as the 'universal intellectual'. However, in Basaglia's work, these intellectuals are not merely spokespersons of a universal knowledge; they are also and especially those who translate this knowledge into a practice of domination: the ruling class exploits intellectuals in order to reinforce its power over the lower classes.

On the other hand, as Robert Castel puts it, the specific intellectual 'remains an intellectual, with all that the term entails in the way of a deontology proper to it'. Yet the specific intellectual must also abandon 'the traditional position of theoretical superiority' (Castel, 1992: 67), insofar as, in Foucault's words, the specific intellectual does not work 'in the modality of the "universal" [...] but within specific sectors'. The localisation of their intervention gives them 'a much more immediate and concrete awareness of struggles' (Foucault, 1986: 68). It is for this reason that specific intellectuals have become closer to the masses, according to Foucault.

When psychiatrists accept the role of specific intellectuals, they can finally provoke a 'crisi pratica di un'ideologia scientifica' (Basaglia, 1975a: 243). That is to say, psychiatrists, acting as specific intellectuals, can unveil the social issues that the scientific ideology of psychiatry masks. In doing so, they are effectively bringing the psychiatric issue to a political level. In Basaglia's (1975a: 246) words, the

> tecnico borghese vive in una condizione di alienazione da cui può uscire rompendo la condizione di oggettivazione in cui vive l'oppresso.

By 'bracketing' mental illness and taking advantage of the inpatient's aggressiveness, psychiatrists can take into account the history and the subjectivity of their former object of study – the patient (Basaglia, 1975a: 246). It is only in this 'ricerca di uno spazio reciproco di soggettivazione' (Basaglia, 1975a: 246), that psychiatrists can effectively oppose the capillary and 'microphysical' dissemination of power in a disciplinary system.[5] Simply put, only a localised struggle can oppose the localised exertion of power.

---

5   Foucault introduced the concept of the 'microphysics of power' in *Psychiatric Power*. During the first lecture, Foucault (2006b: 16) maintains that his course will focus not on violence and institutions but on the 'microphysics of power' that designates 'these immediate, tiny, capillary powers that are exerted on the body, behavior, actions, and time of individuals' (Foucault, 2006b: 16n). Again, in *Discipline and Punish*, Foucault (1991: 139) stresses how the 'meticulous, often minute, techniques [...] had their importance' in defining 'a certain mode of detailed political investment of the body, a new micro-physics of power'. Overall, the concept of the microphysics of power describes the way in which disciplinary power functions: it is a capillary power, exerted on every single individual. It does not need the macrophysics of sovereignty, such as the visibility of the sovereign (in rituals, parades, etc.) or extreme forms

The reforming psychiatrist thus effectively sides with the inmates, much as the engaged, specific, intellectual sides with the lower classes. However, in doing so, in questioning the unbiased nature of the knowledge that guarantees their power over the inmates and in rejecting their social mandate, reforming psychiatrists are 'rejecting their official role' (Donnelly, 1992: 56) and enabling 'the subordinate class to take possession of the technicians' knowledge, and hence emerge themselves as subjects' (Donnelly, 1992: 56). Sartre (1975: 293 also quoted in Basaglia, 1975a: 271) refers precisely to this when he asserts that the 'mission of the intellectual' is to

> suppress himself as an intellectual. What I mean by intellectual, here, is a man with a guilty conscience. What he should learn to do is to put what he has been able to salvage from the disciplines that taught him universal techniques, directly at the service of the masses. Intellectuals must learn to understand the universal that the masses want, in reality, in the immediate, this very moment.

Also, Colucci and Di Vittorio (2001: 219) note that, in Gorizia through the work of deinstitutionalisation, 'muore la figura dell'intellettuale'. Psychiatrists withdraw from their position of power, renounce what is thought of as a pseudo-science that only endorses their discriminating choices, grant the patient the possibility of acting as a subject and finally awaken in the inmate a feeling of rebellion. The suppression of the intellectual as an intellectual and of the psychiatrist as a psychiatrist is aimed at engendering a state of socio-political equality inasmuch as both the psychiatrist and the patient now are regarded as active political subjects, in possession of their basic human rights, with their freedom of expression and so on. But it is also a position of 'phenomenological' and 'existential' equality insofar as, in this condition, psychiatrist and patient eventually enter in the intersubjective authentic 'encounter' Basaglia so keenly argued for during his 'phenomenological' phase: the patient is no longer considered

---

of punishment such as public executions; 'alla trascendenza del sovrano subentra l'immanenza di un governo capace di agire dall'interno sui processi che regola' (De Giorgi, 2006: 121). Disciplinary power works at a local level, almost silently and invisibly, through a capillary, microphysical distribution.

as an object to study, as an anatomical body to move around like furniture, *a priori* labelled as 'sick'.

The Ideological Void: Law 180 and its Aftermath

All these considerations converge in Basaglia's work of deinstitutionalisation in the asylum at Trieste and in the very formulation of the 1978 Law that reshaped psychiatric health care in Italy. Having met the resistance of the local government in Gorizia, Basaglia moved to the Colorno asylum, in Parma, whence he had been invited by the left-wing-led coalition. However, in 1971 he moved again, this time to the asylum at Trieste, since not even the left-wing local authorities in Colorno approved of his revolutionary reforms. In Trieste, initially, Basaglia enforced the reforms he had already carried out in Gorizia: he abolished white coats, physical restraint and shock therapies, opened up the wards and introduced the therapeutic community, all with the aim of humanising psychiatric health care and the life of the inpatients.

From 1973 onwards, after the World Health Organization designated Trieste as a 'pilot zone' for psychiatric health care in Europe, and with the full support of the local government led by Michele Zanetti, Basaglia and his team began to radicalise the efforts of deinstitutionalisation, aiming at emptying the asylum and ultimately closing it down. 1973 saw the approval of the *Cooperativa Lavoratori Uniti*, the first attempt to dignify the work of the inpatients, no longer forced to work with 'ergotherapeutic' aims, but properly employed with legal contracts and represented by a union of their own. Also, in the same year, the parade of the giant blue papier-mâché horse 'Marco Cavallo' took place. Built under the direction of the artist Vittorio Basaglia, Franco's cousin, in one of the former wards of the asylum, the horse was meant to be a symbol of deinstitutionalisation: like a Trojan horse it was meant to carry in its belly the desire and needs of the inpatients outside of the asylum. The sculpture paraded with members of staff and inmates through the main streets of the city of Trieste, raising the awareness of the population with regard to the problems that were formerly locked away in the asylum, to use Mollica's appropriate formulation. Several other initiatives of this kind followed, such as the rental of a holiday house for the inmates in the mountains near Belluno in 1975, and a number of concerts open to the general public inside the walls of the asylum.

In 1974, inspired by the left-wing association 'Magistratura Democratica', Basaglia and his team founded 'Psichiatria Democratica', a group of psychiatrists, nurses and social workers committed to promoting deinstitutionalisation in psychiatry. In 1977, after being weakened by unfavourable local elections, Zanetti's local government had to resign. As time was running out, Basaglia and Zanetti held a press conference and announced that the asylum at Trieste would close by the end of the year. Although they were unable to completely fulfil their declaration, of the 1,200 inpatients of the asylum in 1971, only 130 were still there when Basaglia left Trieste, in 1979.

The *distruzione dell'ospedale psichiatrico* was achieved through the approval of Law 180, hurriedly proposed by the Christian Democrat senator and psychiatrist, Bruno Orsini, and passed in May 1978, to avoid the referendum proposed by the *Radicali*, which would have probably been unsuccessful. Law 180 was included in the final formulation of the new law for public health care on 23 December 1978 (Law 833/1978).[6] Ten years before, another law on public health care had been passed, which had included some articles about psychiatric assistance. Although Law 431/1968 addressed mainly financial issues, it also called into question involuntary hospitalisation. The fourth article added to involuntary psychiatric hospitalisation (*ricovero in regime coatto*) the possibility of patients entering the institution voluntarily. Indirectly, it also created the possibility of turning involuntary hospitalisation into a voluntary stay.[7] Law 36/1904

---

6 Insofar as it relates to psychiatry, Law 883/1978 included the text of Law 180 in its entirety and without any change. For this reason, in this section I will quote only from the text of Law 833/1978, as this is the law currently in force in Italy.

7 *Legge 18 marzo 1968, n. 431, art. 4*. 'La ammissione in ospedale psichiatrico può avvenire volontariamente, su richiesta del malato, per accertamento diagnostico e

had established a direct link between mental illness (at that time referred to as *alienazione mentale*) and social dangerousness, thus effectively stressing the need to protect society from madness. Law 431/1968, known as the *Legge stralcio Mariotti* (from the name of the politician who proposed it), called into question this assumption for the first time. It allowed patients to turn their involuntary hospitalisation into a voluntary admission. This meant that there was no obligation to inform the authorities of an inmate's discharge. Involuntary hospitalisation was not abolished but a new legal category of sickness was created. Mental patients could now partly control their psychiatric treatment and avoid confrontation with public authorities with regard to their illnesses. In other words, these patients were no longer considered dangerous and could actively take part in their therapeutic decisions.

After the *Legge stralcio Mariotti* was passed in 1968, most of the patients in Gorizia were allowed to turn their involuntary hospitalisation into voluntary admission. Thanks to this, by the time Basaglia left Gorizia, most of the inmates of the psychiatric hospital were no longer forced to reside in the asylum.

Arguably, the *Legge stralcio Mariotti* was only a temporary measure, as it merely outlined a new perspective on psychiatric assistance. Italian psychiatric reform proper, that is, the complete abolition of the 1904 law on *alienazione mentale*, was achieved by the inclusion of Law 180 in the general public health care regulation (*Legge 23 Dicembre 1978, n. 833*). Law 180 envisioned three main points of reform: the clear regulation of involuntary hospitalisation, the banning of psychiatric hospitals, the construction of community centres for psychiatric health care.

Articles 33, 34 and 35 of Law 833 decree that involuntary hospitalisation must be enforced 'nel rispetto della dignità della persona e dei diritti

---

cura, su autorizzazione del medico di guardia. In tali casi non si applicano le norme vigenti per le ammissioni, la degenza e le dimissioni dei ricoverati di autorità. La dimissione di persone affette da disturbi psichici ricoverati di autorità, ai sensi delle vigenti disposizioni, negli ospedali psichiatrici è comunicata all'autorità di pubblica sicurezza, ad eccezione dei casi nei quali il ricovero di autorità sia stato trasformato in volontario'. Published in *Gazzetta Ufficiale 20 aprile 1968, n. 101*.

civili e politici' (*Legge 23 Dicembre 1978, n. 833, art. 33, comma 1*) and that the hospitalised person retains the right to 'comunicare con chi ritenga opportuno' (*art. 33, comma 2*) and request an appeal (*art. 33, comma 3*). Also, specifically with regard to psychiatric intervention, involuntary hospitalisation may be enforced only:

> se esistano alterazioni psichiche tali da richiedere urgenti interventi terapeutici, se gli stessi non vengano accettati dall'infermo e se non vi siano le condizioni e le circostanze che consentano di adottare tempestive ed idonee misure sanitare extraospedaliere (*art. 34, comma 4*).

By comparison, the 1904 law had stated that involuntary hospitalisation must be enforced on those people who are 'pericolose a sé o agli altri o riescano di pubblico scandalo e non siano e non possano essere convenientemente custodite e curate fuorché nei manicomi' (*Legge 14 febbraio 1904, n. 36, art. 1, comma 1*). Since 1978, what Law 833 defines as *Trattamento Sanitario Obbligatorio* or 'TSO' (involuntary hospitalisation) has been enforced for the benefit of the sick person and not for the benefit of society. This is a fundamental change in perspective, a 'rivoluzione copernicana' (Colucci and Di Vittorio, 2001: 299), in that it focuses the aims of psychiatric intervention on the individual, rather than on the social body.

Article 64 of Law 833 ratifies what Basaglia (1964a) used to call 'la distruzione dell'ospedale psichiatrico', as it decrees 'il graduale superamento degli ospedali psichiatrici o neuro-psichiatrici e la diversa utilizzazione [...] delle strutture esistenti' (*art. 64, comma 1*). The buildings that housed psychiatric hospitals had to be converted to different purposes, such as offices or, as it happened in Trieste, university campuses.

Law 180 also stipulates that 'è [...] vietato costruire nuovi ospedali psichiatrici' as well as using the existing ones as 'divisioni specialistiche psichiatriche di ospedali generali' (*art. 64, comma 3*). As an alternative to the psychiatric hospital, the new law provided for the creation of local services, in order to guarantee the continuation of psychiatric health care and the support of those in need of assistance. Although the law did not provide for the structure of such centres (to be known as *Centri di Salute Mentale* or 'CSM'), usually they adopted an open-door policy, often on a

24/7 basis. Along with these centres, the law provided for the creation of the *Servizio Psichiatrico di Diagnosi e Cura*, small open-door units of up to fifteen beds in general hospitals, to address acute psychiatric crises and emergencies. In Rotelli's words (1994: 18), Law 180 established

> per la prima volta nella storia dell'umanità, che non debbono più esistere luoghi separati, concentrazionari per i folli.

Despite the revolutionary achievement of this law, Basaglia was far from considering it to be the final act of his work of deinstitutionalisation. As he observed in 'Conversazione: a proposito della Legge 180', Law 180 was a milestone for psychiatric assistance in that it granted mental patients their human rights (Basaglia, 1980). The law finally broke the link between social danger and mental illness. The new legal measures overturned the logic that had governed institutional psychiatry and the asylum ever since the era of the 'great confinement' (Foucault, 2006a: 44), 'that banished madness into the dull, uniform world of exclusion' (Foucault, 2006a: 249). Nevertheless, Basaglia (1980: 470) also noted that 'questa legge ha in qualche modo violentato lo stesso operatore psichiatrico alternativo'. Basaglia's work was entirely structured around the need to reform psychiatry. Once reform was achieved, the anti-institutional psychiatrist had no positive guidelines with which to manage the new, deinstitutionalised system of which he was in charge. Donnelly (1992: 100) regards Basaglia's activism as the positive face of his aversion to producing a psychiatric 'school' or current, grounded on a common theoretical framework: 'the strong activist character of the interventions, [...] was also a cover for a lack of theoretical production'. On the other hand, Lovell and Scheper-Hughes (1987: 4) note that

> Basaglia presented no famous case histories, and no specific therapeutic techniques or practices. Innovations, of course, require new conceptual schemes and reference points, but Basaglia's apprehension that these might freeze into ideological utopias was reminiscent of Sartre's [1948] observation that ideologies are liberating only while they are in the making, and oppressive since they are established.

Also, as Colucci and Di Vittorio (2001: 99) note, the most important outcome of Law 180 was, according to Basaglia, precisely this lack of guidelines. He maintains that this lack of method, technique, guidelines and theories should be regarded as a 'vuoto ideologico' (Basaglia, 1979b: 307). It is a 'momento felice' (Basaglia, 1979b: 307), during which psychiatrists can be independent of the impositions of an implicit ideology, such as biological, institutional or even social psychiatry. When psychiatrists have eventually exhausted their task of dismantling the institution of psychiatry, they can finally deal with mental illness within society as such. In Basaglia's words (1979b: 307),

> disarmati come siamo, privi di strumenti [...] siamo costretti a rapportarci con questa angoscia e questa sofferenza senza oggettivarle automaticamente negli schemi della 'malattia', e senza disporre ancora di un nuovo codice interpretativo che ricreerebbe l'antica istanza fra chi comprende e chi ignora.

The new role of the psychiatrist is to let the subjectivity of the patient emerge, without the mediation of the category of mental illness. The subjectivity of the patient, which had always been Basaglia's primary concern, 'può affiorare solo in un rapporto che [...] riesca a non rinchiudere in una ulteriore oggettivazione l'esperienza abnorme' (Basaglia, 1979b: 307). That is to say, it can emerge in a relationship that is not regulated by *a priori* categorisations.

Yet, as Basaglia's former colleague Agostino Pirella (1987: 133) has remarked, 'merely changing the law is no magic formula for altering the practice of psychiatrists [or] the attitudes of the population'. In a moment of radical changes such as occurred in 1978, psychiatrists are still required to rationalise their work. That is to say, they are required to produce a theory capable of remaking their local work as universal and as objective as possible. As Ongaro Basaglia (1987: 19) observes, 'our culture has tended to resolve things by creating an institution for every phenomenon, for every problem, where all phenomena and problems of the same type can be concentrated'. This holds good also for the alternative psychiatry advocated by Basaglia. The approval of Law 180 thus generates new risks in psychiatry, for instance, the risk of recreating a segregating and stigmatising power inside the newly founded territorial centres. Also, to use Basaglia's words, there is the risk of 'crystallising the answers' to mental illness with a new technique. After the reform, psychiatry ran the risk of being reintegrated within a general system of social control, thus creating new technicians with a newer and more efficient set of 'social' techniques that would serve the same social purpose as institutional psychiatry. It was this outcome Foucault had in mind when he claimed that the destruction of the psychiatric hospital had created a dissemination of power to the small territorial centres that replaced the asylum (Foucault et al., 1994: 664–65). Deinstitutionalisation might have accelerated and prompted the intrusion of psychiatry into everyday life: but, Foucault asks (1994c: 274), is not psychiatry in the community, rather than in the asylum, merely

> une autre façon, plus souple, de faire fonctionner la médecine mentale comme une hygiène publique, présente partout et toujours prête à intervenir?

With this in mind, in the next chapter, I will discuss what happened to psychiatry after the 'destruction' of the asylum. If the biological and institutional psychiatry of the asylum can be related to 'disciplinary' power, in Foucault's terms, then 'deinstitutionalised' psychiatry must be set and analysed against a form of power that, according to Foucault, came into being more recently, and which he calls 'biopolitics'.

CHAPTER 5

Biopolitics and Psychiatry

Introduction

Initially, as we have seen, Foucault described the relationship between madness and reason through the notion of graft. First, in *History of Madness*, he analysed this graft from a historical perspective, from its origins to the age of the asylum. He then addressed the graft's continuation into the twentieth century, when psychiatry became embedded into disciplinary systems. Foucault pursued this reflection during the two decades of the 1960s and 1970s. During those same twenty years, Basaglia fought against the disciplinary power involved in biological and institutional psychiatry as it was then practised in Italy. Foucault and Basaglia did not develop a personal relationship yet their intellectual links in these two decades are evident. Arguably, the tie-ins begin with the opening of the 1964 paper, 'La distruzione dell'ospedale psichiatrico', where Basaglia (1964a: 22) directly refers to the birth of the asylum according to Foucault's *History of Madness*, and continue, though less openly, in Basaglia's study of docile patients and institutionalised bodies – among the effects of disciplinary power, according to Foucault, and in his criticism of the power intrinsic in psychiatry and medicine in general. In 1971, Foucault himself refers to Basaglia for the first time, in an interview that has been extensively studied by Di Vittorio in his 1999 monograph, *Foucault e Basaglia*. Foucault (1994d: 209) says:

> Depuis quelques années s'est développé en Italie, autour de Basaglia, [...] un mouvement [...] ils ont vu dans le livre que j'avais écrit une espèce de justification historique et ils l'ont en quelque sorte réassumé, repris en compte, ils s'y sont, jusqu'à un certain point, retrouvés, et voilà que ce livre historique est en train d'avoir une sorte d'aboutissement pratique. Alors disons que je suis un peu jaloux et que maintenant je voudrais bien faire les choses moi-même.

Di Vittorio equates Foucault's 'jealousy' with Basaglia's later rhetorical question: 'Cosa abbiamo offerto per riflessione alle persone che sventolavano il libretto rosso di Trieste e sul quale non c'era scritto niente' (Balduzzi et al., 1979: 212)?[1] As a consequence Basaglia seems to believe that he and his team should have written 'qualcosa di più in quel libretto rosso'. On the basis of these two quotations, Di Vittorio argues that a reciprocal bond of jealousy links Basaglia and Foucault. Basaglia felt the need to transcend his psychiatric and political practice in order to produce a theoretical work. On the other hand, Foucault seemed to be jealous of the fact that Basaglia transformed his theories into practice. According to Di Vittorio (1999: 15), this is a 'verdetto inequivocabile', as it reveals that 'il filosofo è in crisi, e in preda a gelosia scende per strada'. Foucault apparently discovered that his books would have remained

> muti e vuoti senza quei movimenti di base che, rimettendo praticamente in discussione campi specifici come la psichiatria o la giustizia, rendono possibile un'analisi concreta del potere. (Di Vittorio, 1999: 15–16)

For his part, Basaglia understood that his attempt to reform psychiatry would have been a 'fuoco di paglia fino a quando la negazione del manicomio non verrà vista come un aspetto settoriale di un problema che riguarda la società intera' (Di Vittorio, 1999: 16). Although otherwise limited to a historical and biographical study, Di Vittorio's analysis begins to unearth the complex intellectual relationship between Basaglia and Foucault.

Since they never met in person, the most probable intermediary between Foucault and Basaglia was the French sociologist Robert Castel,

---

1   Basaglia is here referring to Mao's *Red Book*. Ever since the 1960s, the phrase 'sventolare il libretto rosso' has derogatorily indicated the act of publicly defending an ideology without a background understanding of its implications. Basaglia is here openly criticising both himself and those who supported his work. As he seems to imply, these supporters would have backed his work without questioning that they were in fact adhering to an ideology and not subscribing to a consistent philosophy. As a matter of fact, Basaglia seems to suggest that he did not offer enough theoretical grounds to his supporters, who often ended up 'waving his *Red Book*', in which nothing was written.

director of the *École des hautes études en sciences sociales* at the time of writing. Castel met Basaglia at a conference in Paris in 1968, and decided to visit Gorizia, where they established a lifelong intellectual collaboration. Castel (2005: 13) is very clear on this: Basaglia, he says, 'è stato probabilmente l'uomo più importante della mia vita'. It was thanks to Castel's mediation that Basaglia's edited collection *Crimini di pace* (1975) could include Foucault's 'La casa della follia', which, later, turned out to be a modified version of the resumé of his course, *Psychiatric Power*. Most probably, it was through Castel that Basaglia followed Foucault's two courses at the *Collége de France*, dedicated to psychiatry (*Le Pouvoir psychiatrique*, 1973–74, and *Les Anormaux*, 1974–75), since their proceedings have only recently been published in French and Italian.[2] However, their conclusions concerning disciplinary power, its connection to psychiatry, and the expansion of discipline beyond enclosed institutions converge with Foucault's analysis of sovereignty, discipline, and punishment in *Surveiller et punir* (*Discipline and Punish*), which was published in French in 1975, and translated into Italian soon after (1976). In 1977, a very important collection of essays by Foucault was published in Italian. It was entitled *Microfisica del potere*, and included, among other texts, 'Nietzsche: La généalogie, l'histoire' ('Nietzsche, Genealogy and History'), 'Au de là du bien et du mal' ('Beyond Good and Evil') and the first two lectures of the 1975–76 course *Il faut défendre la societé* (*Society Must Be Defended*). Hence, although many key texts by Foucault were still unpublished, Basaglia certainly had wide access to his ideas.

2   *Les Anormaux* edited by Ewald, Fontana, Marchetti, and Salomoni, was published by Seuil-Gallimard in 1999; the Italian edition, translated by Marchetti and Salomoni was published by Feltrinelli in 2000, under the title *Gli anormali* and the English edition, translated by Burchell, was published by Picador in 2003, under the title *Abnormal*. *Le Pouvoir psychiatrique*, edited by Lagrange, Ewald, Fontana, and Snellart, was not published until 2003, also by Seuil-Gallimard; the English edition, translated by Burchell was published by Palgrave MacMillan in 2006 under the title *Psychiatric Power* and the Italian edition, translated by Bertani, was published by Feltrinelli in 2004, under the title *Il potere psichiatrico*.

Similarly, during the 1970s, Foucault became more aware of Basaglia and his work, which he always associated with the anti-psychiatric current (he also includes the American Szasz and the British Laing and Cooper in that). As I pointed out in the conclusion to the previous chapter, there are a number of published interviews and roundtables during which Foucault expressly refers to Basaglia – and I will return to them in due course in this chapter. In the *resumé* of the course on psychiatric power, Foucault also refers to numerous 'anti-psychiatric' experiences, such as Cooper's Villa 21, Laing and Cooper's Kingsley Hall, and the asylum in Gorizia. 'Power relations, he says, were the *a priori* of psychiatric practice: they conditioned how the asylum institution functioned, they determined the distribution of relationships between individuals within it, and they governed the forms of medical intervention'. However, in those places employing 'anti-psychiatry', power relations were placed 'at the center of the problematic field [...] questioning them in a fundamental way' (Foucault, 2006b: 345). In several other places, however, Foucault seemed much more sceptical about the revolutionary reach of anti-psychiatry (for instance, Foucault, 1994c).

I will return in due course to these instances. It is now time to discuss how 'disciplinary psychiatry', i.e. the 'first biological psychiatry' (Shorter, 1997: 69) as it was practised within the walls of the asylum, evolves. If this medical approach to madness could easily be defined in terms of Foucault's disciplinary power, its dismantling, which Basaglia carried out in Gorizia, Colorno, Trieste, and the implementation of Law 180, seemed to pave the way for a different form of psychiatry, which could be described in terms of Foucault's disciplinary society first and then biopolitics. After having introduced these, in this chapter, I analyse how such notions can be applied to psychiatry. Particular attention is given to psychiatry as it is practised today, therefore a brief introduction is given on its main epistemological, clinical and epidemiological implications, and their connections with political praxis and governance of the population, worldwide and in the Italian context. This leads therefore to concluding with a discussion of how Basaglia commented on psychiatry after Law 180, and how his 'heirs' harshly criticised the rise of a 'biopolitical psychiatry', ascribing to it an aura that is exclusively negative and coercive.

Disciplinary Society, Biopolitics and Biopower

In Foucault's work, the first occurrence of the term 'biopolitics' can be traced back to a paper delivered at a conference in Brazil in 1974, entitled *Crisis de un modelo en la medicina?* This paper has been published in Portuguese with this title (Foucault, 1976a) and translated into Spanish with the title *La crisis de la medicina o la crisis de la anti-medicina* (Foucault, 1976b). While the French and Italian translations (Foucault, 1994a, 1997a) are based on the Portuguese text, the English one (Foucault, 2004) is based on the Spanish translation. Neither the Spanish nor the English text contains any reference to the concept of bio-politics. The Italian translation, however, contains the following: 'per la società capitalistica è il bio-politico a essere importante prima di tutto, il biologico, il somatico, il corporale. Il corpo è una realtà bio-politica; la medicina è una strategia politica' (Foucault, 1997a: 222).

Certainly, as Lemke, in his *Biopolitics: An Advanced Introduction* (2011), correctly shows, 'biopolitics' is not a concept introduced by Foucault but by Rudolph Kjellen in 1920 (Kjellen, 1920: 93–94). However, Foucault's is the longest-lasting and most influential of its definitions. Before Foucault, 'biopolitics' was used either with a 'naturalistic' inflection 'that take[s] life as the basis of politics' or with a 'politicist' inflection, 'which conceive[s] of life processes as the object of politics' (Lemke, 2011: 3): either life shapes politics (for instance, regarding society as an organism, applying notions such as the survival of the fittest to the socio-political context, and so on), or politics shapes life (for instance managing the health of the population, natality, morbidity and mortality, and so on).

Foucault (2003b: 242) somehow overcame this distinction, as I will show, by proposing to describe biopolitics as 'a new technology of power', which does not rule out disciplinary power but 'integrates it, modifies it [...] and uses it [...] by embedding itself in existing disciplinary techniques'. The boundaries between discipline and biopolitics, however, are blurred, and it seems to me that Foucault intended them to be so: biopolitics evolves from disciplinary techniques; it embeds and overcomes them. Foucault seemed to regard the chronological transition between sovereignty and biopolitics as a four-stage process: sovereign power; discipline inside the institutions (e.g. asylums); disciplinary society, when disciplinary power is no longer limited by the walls of the enclosed institutions and invests the whole of society; and, finally, biopolitics. Although Foucault does identify the historical origins of some of these forms of power, he has never been clear on their chronological boundaries, with the possible implication that all forms of power (sovereign, disciplinary inside the institution, disciplinary society and even biopolitics) can coexist, to different extents, with one dominant form, in different places and at different times.

In *Psychiatric Power*, Foucault maintains that 'disciplinary power [...] has a history; it is not born suddenly, has not always existed'. Although disciplinary power 'was not completely marginal to medieval society', instances of it are limited and generally only occur 'within religious communities'. The birth of disciplinary power can be pinned down to a 'symbolic reference point', which is, according to Foucault (2006b: 40–41), 'when [it] becomes an absolutely generalized social form [...] in 1791, with Bentham's *Panopticon*'. Also in *Discipline and Punish*, Foucault (1991: 137) observes that although 'many disciplinary methods had long been in existence', there is a point in history during which 'one can speak of the formation of a disciplinary society' (Foucault, 1991: 216). This moment is when Bentham's *panopticon* – an enclosed institution – becomes 'an indefinitely generalizable mechanism of "panopticism"' (Foucault, 1991: 216). Most of the disciplinary techniques 'have a long history behind them'; nevertheless, in the eighteenth century, 'by being combined and generalized, they attained a level at which the formation of knowledge and the increase of power regularly reinforce one another in a circular process' (Foucault, 1991: 224) Disciplinary power produces individuality, in that, through a series of exercises, under constant supervision, abiding by a number of norms, people subject themselves – without the actual need for someone to wield power – to a certain notion of individuality and subjectivity. They are under the spell of power even when there is no supervisor; they end up disciplining themselves. This form of power pervades society in its entirety when it overflows the walls of institutions such as asylums, schools and prisons: this is the beginning of disciplinary society.

It is unclear in *Discipline and Punish* whether Foucault considers 'disciplinary society' as a stage that follows chronologically the rise of discipline in enclosed institutions. Statements such as 'one can speak of the formation of a disciplinary society in this movement that stretches from the enclosed disciplines' (Foucault, 1991: 216) imply at least that the rise of discipline in enclosed institutions precedes that of a disciplinary society.

However, what is clear is that this is not yet 'biopolitics', strictly speaking. Biopolitics embeds disciplinary power and grows on top of and through disciplinary society, but it entails a much more systematic and statistical approach: the object of biopolitics is no longer the single individual, but the population, the mass of single subjects statistically normalised into the perfect individual, the perfect object of power. And what biopolitics targets about individuals is their anatomical body, their biological lives, not only in terms of discipline – e.g. exercises to normalise the bodily functions, make the body visible to the supervisor, address concerns of personal hygiene, etc. – but also and especially in terms of population: biopolitics addresses the statistics of morbidity and mortality, matters of epidemiology, nationwide campaigns of disease prevention, birth rates, etc. Biopolitics, in Foucault's terms (2008b: 317), is 'the attempt, starting from the eighteenth century, to rationalize the problems posed to governmental practice by phenomena characteristic of a set of living beings forming a population: health, hygiene, birthrate, life expectancy, race.' Biopolitics, all things considered, is the governance of the anatomical bodies of the population, the governance of the social body understood in biological terms.

To a certain extent, biopolitics overcomes the tension between individuality and multiplicity that disciplinary power could not solve. Discipline 'is addressed to bodies' (Foucault, 2003b: 242), in that it aims at controlling individual bodies as distinct from the mass, i.e. the multiplicity of individuals they may constitute. Discipline individualises insofar as the formation of a mass is the biggest threat to its power. Biopolitics, on the other hand, has, as its object, the 'global mass' of individuals, insofar as they can be all reduced to their shared organic and mental processes (Foucault, 2003b: 242). If the disciplinary 'seizure of power over the body is an individualizing move', the power that biopolitics exerts 'is not individualizing but [...] massifying' (Foucault, 2003b: 243). Biopolitics does not rule out disciplinary power: it exploits disciplinary techniques by rationalising and systematising their application.

However, several scholars, among them Esposito (2004: 27), problematise a possible linear understanding of the evolution of power according to Foucault, not only in reference to the relationship between discipline and biopolitics, but also and especially in reference to sovereignty/biopolitics: 'Foucault si astiene dal fornire una risposta definitiva [su come] si rapportano sovranità e biopolitica'. For instance, in *Society Must Be Defended*, Foucault (2003b: 35–36) seems to believe that discipline is a 'new mechanism of power', which is 'the exact, point-for-point opposite of the mechanics of power' of sovereignty. In the first volume of *History of Sexuality*, Foucault (1998: 138) argues that biopolitics evolves from discipline when it completely replaces the very grounds of sovereignty: 'the ancient right to *take* life or *let* live was replaced by a power to *foster* life or *disallow* it to the point of death'. Yet, in this definition of biopolitics as the power that both *fosters* and *disallows* life, Foucault's 'ambivalences', as Bazzicalupo (2010: 62) calls them, emerge.

Foucault has never been particularly clear in distinguishing between the aspect of biopolitics that *fosters* life and that which *disallows* it, nor between the notion of biopolitics and the related concept of 'biopower' (see, for instance, Lemke, 2011: 34). In Esposito's words, Foucault 'non ha mai articolato a sufficienza il concetto di politica – al punto da sovrapporre sostanzialmente le espressioni di "biopotere" e "biopolitica"' (Esposito, 2004: 39). Rabinow and Rose try to resolve this ambiguity by defining biopower(s) as the 'more or less rationalized attempts to intervene upon the vital characteristics' of human beings, considered 'as living creatures who are born, mature, inhabit a body that can be trained and augmented, and then sicken and die', and also of 'collectives and populations composed of such living beings' (Rabinow and Rose, 2006: 196–97). On the other hand, they define biopolitics as those 'specific strategies and contestations over problematizations of collective human vitality, morbidity and mortality; over the forms of knowledge, regimes of authority and practices of intervention that are desirable, legitimate and efficacious' (Rabinow and Rose, 2006: 197). It could be said that, whereas biopower is the power exerted on the population, when this is understood as a collective of biological bodies, biopolitics is the organisation and systematisation of such power by the political forces that govern these collectives. Nevertheless, Rabinow and Rose (2006: 197) also agree that Foucault is 'somewhat imprecise in his use of terms' and they regret that there has been no systematic study of his 'sketchy suggestions' on biopolitics and biopower.

If fostering life, by protecting and enhancing it, is arguably very different from the idea of a sovereign's limiting life, through impositions, taxes, capital punishment, and so on, the possibility of *disallowing* life seems to converge with the sovereign's right of life and death over the subjects. This contradiction is already evident in *Society Must Be Defended*, where Foucault states that the new power is on all points the exact opposite of sovereignty but also contends that:

> I wouldn't say exactly that sovereignty's old right – to take life or let live – was replaced but it came to be complemented by a new right which does not erase the old right but which does penetrate it, permeate it. (Foucault, 2003b: 241)

In different ways, both Esposito and Agamben try to resolve this contradiction by distinguishing between a modulation of biopolitics that does indeed *foster* life and one that *disallows* it, which they both call 'thanatopolitics'. Yet, biopolitics and thanatopolitics are two sides of the same coin, because they rest, to put it bluntly, on the same premise that political power can and should somehow systematically interfere with the very biological life of every single individual.

Esposito distinguishes between a *politica della vita* and a *politica sulla vita*. The *politica della vita* could be regarded as an affirmative biopolitics, which 'fosters life', 'in contrasto con l'attitudine impositiva del regime sovrano' (Esposito, 2004: 31). While sovereignty 'si esercitava in termini di sottrazione, di prelievo', this affirmative biopolitics

> si rivolge alla vita non soltanto nel senso della sua difesa, ma anche in quello del suo dispiegamento, del suo potenziamento, della sua massimizzazione. (Esposito, 2004: 30)

On the other hand, a *politica sulla vita* corresponds to the 'sviluppo del biopotere e incremento della capacità omicida' (Esposito, 2004: 33), which he calls *thanatopolitics*. This aspect of biopolitics is not a break from but a continuity of sovereignty in that it is marked by the return of the 'antico potere sovrano di dare la morte' (Esposito, 2004: 36): biopolitics and biopower do not only foster life but they can also disallow it.

According to Agamben (2005: 9), sovereignty and biopolitics are intrinsically connected. He believes that 'l'implicazione della nuda vita nella sfera politica costituisce il nucleo originario – anche se occulto – del potere sovrano'. In other words, there has never been such a thing as a sovereign power that is not always-already biopolitical, as Foucault, at times, seems to suggest. In Agamben's words, '*si può dire, anzi, che la produzione di un corpo biopolitico sia la prestazione originale del potere sovrano*' (Agamben, 2005: 9; original emphasis). The intrinsically biopolitical nucleus of all western politics lies in the notion of *homo sacer*, which he draws from ancient Roman law. The *homines sacri*, literally 'sacred men', were not sacred in the current common understanding of the term; they were 'set apart', banned, stripped of their civil rights and cast out of society. While this could be seen as a destiny similar to that met by the inmate in the asylum described by Foucault in *Psychiatric Power*, there are two crucial characteristics of the *homo sacer* that distinguish it from the inmate: first, anyone who had been declared *homo sacer* could be killed with impunity; secondly, the *homo sacer* could not be sacrificed in a religious ritual. For Agamben, this double characteristic brings forth the notion of *nuda vita* or 'bare life', a life that is directly implicated with political power in the form of an 'esclusione inclusiva' (Agamben, 2005: 10). In other words, this bare life is 'inclusa nell'ordinamento unicamente nella forma della sua esclusione (cioè della sua assoluta uccidibilità)' (Agamben, 2005: 12). The sovereign's power to declare someone a *homo sacer*; that is to say, to strip someone of all rights and reduce one to a bare life that can be eliminated without murder being committed, is for Agamben the original biopolitical character of sovereignty, that characteristic which makes all forms of western politics biopolitical to a certain extent. Nonetheless, a critical change took place in the twentieth century that engendered a drift from biopolitics into *thanatopolitics*: the absolute power to *disallow* life. Such, for instance, was the Nazi *Euthanasie-Programm*:

> Se al sovrano [...] compete in ogni tempo il potere di decidere quale vita possa essere uccisa senza commettere omicidio, nell'età della biopolitica questo potere tende ad emanciparsi [...] in potere di decidere sul punto in cui la vita cessa di essere politicamente rilevante. (Agamben, 2005: 157)

In the notion of *homo sacer*, Agamben summarises the intrinsic power of any political system to discriminate between those lives that are allowed to live and those that can be eliminated without consequences (bare lives). The Nazi *Euthanasie-Programm* brought this discrimination to its extremity, in that

> si colloca [...] all'incrocio fra la decisione sovrana sulla vita uccidibile e l'assunzione della cura del corpo biologico della nazione, e segna il punto in cui la biopolitica si rovescia necessariamente in tanatopolitica. (Agamben, 2005: 157)

By virtue of being grounded in the same, ageless notion of *homo sacer*, biopolitics and thanatopolitics (i.e. the fostering and the disallowing of life by means of political power) are two sides of the same coin, and the former constantly runs the risk of turning into the latter.

More than trying to solve the contradiction between affirmative biopolitics and biopower, biopolitics and thanatopolitics, the politics *of* life and politics *over* life, it is important to understand how these considerations on biopolitics can be applied to psychiatry, especially in the Italian post-Basaglian context. It is with this aim in mind that, in the next section, I analyse the concept of 'biopolitical psychiatry' as a possible evolution of early twentieth century disciplinary psychiatry.

Biopolitical Psychiatry

According to Di Vittorio (2006: 73), 'biopolitical psychiatry', which adopts 'an apparatus of prevention' and 'classifies, pathologizes, and institutionalizes a much larger segment of the population', emerges from disciplinary psychiatry as it was practised in the asylum. Its roots can be traced back to the convergence of psychiatry and the judicial system in their common definition of 'abnormality'. Di Vittorio's analysis is profoundly indebted to Foucault's *Abnormal* (2003a), in which he describes how psychiatry became a medico-legal expertise, entrusted with the assessment of the behaviour of entire segments of the population. This new psychiatric knowledge was ultimately aimed at explaining 'scientifically "who" the criminal was' (Di Vittorio, 2006: 77); that is, it was meant to anticipate and prevent crime by spotting dangerousness in the everyday conduct of individuals. As we have seen, this alleged potential dangerousness was identified with abnormality, and it was through this identification that psychiatry ceased to study exclusively the disorders of the mind, in order to address the totality of the 'inner space of the individual', which thus became the 'privileged object of psychiatric gaze' (Rose, 2007: 194). In other words, by becoming the 'scienza e tecnica di gestione delle anomalie' it turned into an 'istanza generale di difesa della società contro i pericoli che la corrodono dall'interno' (Bertani, 2004: 61).

It is precisely this possible evolution that may have been overlooked by psychiatrists after Basaglia. As Di Vittorio (2006: 75) suggests, 'reformed Italian psychiatry has failed to recognize that the new "mental health" policy is biopolitical as well'. Colucci agrees with Di Vittorio on this point and, as he writes in the recent article, 'Scienza del pericolo, clinica del deficit', this is precisely the 'rischio biopolitico che corrono molti operatori psichiatrici'. Psychiatric workers are asked to take over control of the sick person in order to enforce a social order that has not changed since the era of the asylum (Colucci, 2008: 113). Despite Basaglia's reform, Italian psychiatry 'non ha potuto mettere tra parentesi del tutto la medicalizzazione della sofferenza' (Colucci, 2008: 111), which is ultimately the 'riduzione in malattia di tutti i bisogni' of the psychiatric patient (Colucci, 2008: 112). Both Colucci and Di Vittorio seem sceptical about the ultimate outcome of psychiatric reforms, which they deem to be only partially successful, however revolutionary.

More generally, Foucault himself had some reservations on the positive effects of the 1960s–1970s wave of reformism in psychiatry. Initially, Foucault praised the achievements of the anti-psychiatrists, among whom he expressly listed Basaglia, along with Szasz and Cooper (2006b: 345–46). Foucault (2006b: 342) regarded anti-psychiatry as

> everything that calls into question the role of the psychiatrist previously given responsibility for producing the truth of illness within the hospital space.

Anti-psychiatric movements seemed to give 'the individual the task and right of taking his madness to the limit'. Notably, these movements were able to demedicalise madness, therefore freeing the patients 'from the diagnosis and symptomatology' (Foucault, 2006b: 346).

In 1977, Foucault reassessed anti-psychiatry, and his opinion became more cautious. It seemed to him that anti-psychiatry had not been able to oppose the fact that, ever since the nineteenth century, 'nous sommes tous devenus psychiatrisables' (Foucault, 1994c: 273). He went on to question whether practising a form of psychiatry that could work outside the confines of the asylum was actually a break with nineteenth-century psychiatry and whether anti-psychiatry was not a subtler way of making medicine work in the interest of public hygiene by being always present and ready to intervene (Foucault, 1994c: 274). While he was directly referring to the French experience of sectorial psychiatry and institutional psychotherapy, his remarks can be seamlessly applied to Italy. The reform of psychiatry may have effectively pulled down the walls of the asylum: to this extent, it can be considered successful, as it achieved the transformation and eventual abandonment of the disciplinary techniques that were practised first inside the asylum, and then in the reformed and humanised psychiatric hospital. Yet, Foucault queries whether this had not in fact resulted in a generalised psychiatrisation of everyday life. The psychiatrist Hassoun summarised this point at a round table on psychiatric expertise in which Foucault participated: 'il n'y a plus les murs de l'asile. Ils ont éclaté. Ils englobent la ville' (Foucault et al., 1994: 665). Marine Zecca, a sociologist and Cooper's former collaborator, expressed her doubts concerning the Italian psychiatric reform with a similar question: 'hasn't one simply broken up the hospital into tiny external centres that play the same role – that of confinement?' (Cooper et al., 1988: 198). Even if 'l'internamento coatto a vita' is no longer enforced, it has been allegedly substituted for by 'nuovi procedimenti di emarginazione, [...] meno violenti e appariscenti' (Berlincioni and Petrella, 2008: 109). This state of affairs could be legitimately regarded as psychiatry being practised in what Foucault called the 'disciplinary society'.

Foucault distinguishes two main stages in the evolution of psychiatric power. The first amounts to the medicalisation of psychiatry inside the asylum, which results in a new medical science entrusted with the control of dangerous deviants, on the basis that their dangerousness and madness can be ascribed to their organic body. According to Foucault, medicine at this stage is simply a guarantor of psychiatric knowledge and allows psychiatry to function as a disciplinary power, the discipline of disciplines. At the second stage, psychiatry ceases to be the science of 'aliens', those suffering from a mental disorder; it 'dis-alienises' itself, by becoming the science of conduct and behaviour. This brings about a more generalised medicalisation: psychiatry functions as a form of public hygiene, which both controls dangerous deviants, and preventively detects all possible dangerousness (and madness). Di Vittorio regards this stage as the beginning of 'biopolitical' psychiatry, and I would partially agree, at least to the extent that it is indeed on the basis of the disciplinary society that biopolitics, understood in Foucault's terms, first gains a foothold in western society.

Anti-psychiatrists may have played a key role in reinforcing the medicalisation of daily life. A third stage in the evolution of psychiatric power emerges, involving the capillary medicalisation and psychiatrisation of all individuals, sane and insane. It is this stage that sanctions the 'trionfo generalizzato di tutto ciò che ha validità neuroscientifica, reale o presunta' (Colucci, 2008: 115); a renewal of the interest in the organic body (Husserl's *Körper*) to the detriment of what Basaglia, among others, referred to as the 'corpo vissuto' (Husserl's *Leib*). On the other hand, what remains of social and community intervention is still grounded on 'modelli di riabilitazione', which is just another term for 'tecniche di adattamento alla normalità'. These techniques exploit 'moduli di addestramento e assistenze invalidanti, che non sanno che farsene della specificità del soggetto' and still conceal the 'vecchie forme di tutela della società dal folle' (Colucci, 2008: 115).

On the one hand, therefore, what is imputed to the reforms of psychiatry carried out during the 1960s and 1970s is that they did reinforce the link between psychiatry and medicine, reaffirming the medical nature of psychiatric interventions and thus the organic origins of mental illness. On the other hand, critics have focused on the widespread psychiatrisation of everyday life, which eventually brought us to understand ourselves, our moods, feelings, behaviour and reactions more and more in psychiatric terms. However, this cannot yet be regarded, strictly speaking, as 'biopolitical': a shift must be identified that brings systematisation and rationalisation at a governmental level to those features that could otherwise still be ascribed to an 'old' disciplinary regime, albeit no longer enclosed in the institution, but spread into a 'disciplinary society'.

Critics such as Di Vittorio or Colucci seem to have a clear and unambiguous definition of 'biopolitical psychiatry', a psychiatry practised in a biopolitical regime, as opposed to the old, institutionalised disciplinary psychiatry. Equally clearly, they seem to understand biopolitical psychiatry as an unwanted side effect of reformism in psychiatry, a negative drift that could and should have been prevented. If the reform was aimed at dismantling an institutional psychiatry, based, loosely put, on disciplinary apparatuses, it cannot be regarded as completely successful, insofar as it did not prevent the rise of a biopolitical psychiatry which is regarded as a continuation of the former practice. Similarly, they seem to regard biopolitical psychiatry as a betrayal of Basaglia's legacy. Before delving deeper to assess these claims, it is necessary to summarise the current state of psychiatry, in order to have a better notion of how psychiatry is practised today, its epistemological foundations, its clinical approaches and outcomes, and also its macro-social ramifications, such as epidemiological studies and the promotion of mental health. This overview will allow me to give a better picture of what 'biopolitical psychiatry' is now or, at least, what it means to practise psychiatry under biopolitical conditions.

The 'Second Biological Psychiatry'

In his *History of Psychiatry*, Shorter (1997: 239*ff*) refers to contemporary psychiatry as the 'second biological psychiatry'. We have seen that, since its definition as a medical specialty at the beginning of the nineteenth century, psychiatry has sought a connection with the biological body. However, its first attempts were rather clumsy and bore few clinical results: no effective physical treatment was discovered before the advent of the first psychopharmaceuticals (arguably, with the exception of the much-contested electroconvulsive therapy), and no organic aetiology or pathogenesis for mental illness was found. According to Shorter (1997: 145*ff*), the failed attempts of the first biological psychiatry brought about a pessimism that resulted in a dominance – at least outside of Italy – of psychodynamic and psychosocial models of mental illness, relying on 'talk therapies' as the preferred treatment and on psychodynamic (especially psychoanalytical) concepts for assessment and diagnosis. The second *Diagnostic and Statistical Manual of Mental Disorders* (DSM-II), published in 1968 (APA, 1968), precursor of the current 'bible' of psychiatric diagnosis, the DSM-IV – soon to be followed by the DSM-V – relied heavily on psychoanalytical and psychodynamic notions, such as unresolved family conflicts, childhood traumas and so on.

As new, biologically oriented, research began to bear more promising results, what Shorter (1997: 145) called the 'psychoanalytical hiatus' began to close, giving rise to the second biological psychiatry (see also Andreasen, 1997), and the resurgence of the hypothesis of an organic aetiopathogenesis of mental illness. Several studies contributed to this shift in perspective, focusing on issues such as genetics, new imaging techniques and biochemical analyses of neurotransmitters. Although this might change in time, the first two found little to no application in clinical practice: there are no genes unequivocally associated with specific mental illnesses and 'localized brain activity is just as likely to be a result of mental activity as it is to be a cause of it' (Paris, 2008: 16).

The studies on neurotransmitters, on the contrary, found wider applications in clinical practice. In the past, very little was known about how neurones communicated with each other, and the dominant theory was that synapses exchanged electric signals. More recently, it has been discovered that neurones interact also chemically rather than only electrically: the 'chemical messengers' – compounds that derive mainly from amino-acids – between neurones have been called neurotransmitters. The most abundant of these neurotransmitters is glutamate but that most central to psychiatry is serotonin (a hormone otherwise known as 5-Hydroxytryptamine), whose action is associated with a wide range of psychological reactions, states and moods (such as excitement, appetite, sleep regulation, etc.), and whose deficiency is hypothesised to be associated with a number of mental disorders such as depression and anxiety (Carver and Miller, 2006). This, however, has never been completely confirmed by research (Valenstein, 1998).

In spite of the undeniable progress in biochemical research, 'for most mental health problems the aetiology is not fully known', and the panorama is still dominated by so-called 'functional' disorders; that is to say, non-organic: schizophrenia, depression, anxiety, and so forth. The causes of mental illnesses are likely to be 'multiple and heterogeneous' and the most reasonable model of psychiatric aetiopathogenesis is the 'biopsychosocial' one: mental disorders are caused by an overlapping of biological factors (e.g. heredity, natal hazards, physical and neurological diseases, poisoning, etc.), psychological factors (e.g. traumas, low self-esteem, etc.) and social factors (e.g. unemployment, divided families, social disintegration, low social support, etc.) (Lehtinen et al., 2007: 127).

Consequently, diagnosis in psychiatry is still rather uncertain, to the point that Paris (2008: 39) can affirm that 'unlike well-defined diagnoses in other fields of medicine, only a few psychiatric diagnoses have been fully validated; the rest are makeshifts in the absence of something better'. The central problem in psychiatry is the complete absence of biological markers for mental illness (see also Singh and Rose, 2009): there is no lab test, blood test, MRI or CAT scan that can establish which mental illness one is suffering from, or even, for that matter, whether one suffers from a mental illness at all. The absence of biomarkers is not the only problem that psychiatrists face in diagnosis. Physicians from other specialties do diagnose on the basis of sign and symptom observation before seeking confirmation in lab tests. However, diagnosis is usually categorised on the basis of the aetiology of the disease (what *causes* it) or in its pathogenesis (*how* it begins and develops). Yet, for mental illness, neither the aetiology nor the pathogenesis are usually known: most psychiatric disorders have either unknown or numerous and diverse causes and the process that leads to the development of symptoms is equally obscure. Hence, as Paris (2008: 40) correctly notes, mental illnesses are not *diseases* in a medical sense, but *syndromes*; that is to say, a collection of signs (observable pathologic phenomena) and symptoms (subjectively perceived pathologic phenomena) that, in a majority of cases, occur together. This does not mean, however, that they have necessarily emerged from a common cause or through the same process.

> The main motivation behind current practice is that psychiatrists do not want to be isolated from medicine. They want to be like other physicians. This helps explain why the profession has taken up diagnosis so enthusiastically. We want to believe we can diagnose patients accurately and prescribe treatment specific to these categories. However, with our present knowledge, these beliefs are unjustified. Although diagnosis is a necessary tool for psychiatry, the categories we use are not as real as those of stroke or tuberculosis. We may be able to establish scientifically valid diagnoses in the future, but our current knowledge is insufficient to allow us to do so. (Paris, 2008: 41)

Yet, even in general parlance psychiatric diagnoses such as depression, generalised anxiety disorder (GAD), post-traumatic stress disorder (PTSD), attention deficit and hyperactivity disorder (ADHD) and so forth, do proliferate. Given the above considerations it is legitimate to ask ourselves where these diagnoses come from. As I briefly discussed in the first chapter, by the end of the nineteenth century some monumental nosologies of psychiatry had appeared, the most famous and influential of which was certainly Kraepelin's. This nosology based its categorisation on groupings of signs and symptoms, not unlike the most recent psychiatric diagnostic manuals, whose first editions were in fact based on Kraepelin's work. Today, two texts are most influential and their classification of mental illnesses is, by and large, comparable. These are the DSM–IV–TR, the revision of the fourth edition of the *Diagnostic and Statistical Manual of Mental Disorders* (by the American Psychiatric Association, revised in 2000), and the ICD–10, the tenth edition of the *International Statistical Classification of Diseases and Related Health Problems*, by the World Health Organization, which, in Chapter V, lists 'Mental and Behavioural Disorders' (it includes disorders with organic roots (F00–F09), substance-related abuses (F10–F19), affective (F30–F39), neurotic (F40–F48), physiologically related (F50–F59), personality (F60–F69), developmental (F80–F89) and behavioural (F90–F98) disorders).

Biopolitics and Psychiatry 153

Both manuals rely on a rather simple approach – derogatorily called the 'Chinese menu' (Rigier, 2007: S3): to ascertain the presence of a certain disorder the psychiatrist has to observe a certain number of signs and symptoms from a selection of possible indicators.

A simple example, to pick one beyond the commonly cited depressive disorders, would be 'oppositional defiant disorder' (DSM code 313.81), which can be diagnosed if the (young) patient presents four or more of the following symptoms, for more than six months and more frequently than 'typically observed in individuals of comparable age and developmental level', producing clinically significant social/academic/occupational impairment (APA, 2000: 102):

1 often loses temper;
2 often argues with adults;
3 often actively defies or refuses to comply with adults' requests or rules;
4 often deliberately annoys people;
5 often blames others for his or her mistakes or misbehaviour;
6 is often touchy or easily annoyed by others;
7 is often angry and resentful;
8 is often spiteful or vindictive.

Of course, as Paris (2008: 84) does not fail to note, such 'diagnosis is based on observations of behavior that can often be subjective, guided by DSM–IV criteria that are themselves imprecise. And when the boundaries are fuzzy, over-diagnosis becomes a danger'.

The DSM–IV–TR also offers, for each diagnosable syndrome, specific age and gender features, prevalence (which, in epidemiological terms is the percentage of individuals affected in relation to those at risk), course (possible ramifications and development of the disorder), familial pattern (in statistical terms the characteristics of the family in which the individual is more likely to develop the disorder) and finally, guidelines for differential diagnosis. The DSM–IV–TR does not offer any guidelines as regards the treatment of the diagnosed disorders. Also, as First (2005) notes, the DSM–IV–TR prompts for co-morbid diagnoses; that is to say, for assigning two or more simultaneous diagnoses to patients, often disregarding the likely connection between the different disorders (Paris, 2008: 45). For instance, as Goldberg and Goodyer (2005) show, depression and anxiety are a common diagnosis of co-morbidity, although it is likely that they derive from the same process.

Murray and Lopez (1996) show that in 1990 psychiatric and neurological disorders combined accounted for 10 per cent of disability and premature death worldwide. This percentage increased to 12.9 per cent in 2002 and is expected to reach 15 per cent by 2020 (Murray and Lopez 1996). More recently, a survey conducted by Kessler et al. (2005) led them to the conclusion that about half of the entire American population experiences at least one DSM–IV–TR diagnosable psychiatric episode in their lifetime. Studies on prevalence and epidemiology are flourishing in psychiatry; a statistically significant portion of the population has been found to be suffering or have suffered from a mental illness, and the amount is seemingly bound to increase with time. In fact, according to the numerous epidemiological studies, mental disorders are increasingly common (Goldberg and Huxley, 1980; 1992; Bland et al., 1994; Kessler et al., 1994; Meltzer et al., 1995; Almeida-Filho et al., 1997; Bijl et al., 1998; Andrews et al., 2001; Jacobi et al., 2004; Kessler et al., 2005; Pirkola et al., 2005) and from these it can be concluded that about 50 per cent of the general population has suffered or will suffer from a mental disorder in their lifetime (Lehtinen et al., 2007: 128).

This raises a number of legitimate questions; for example, Carey (2005a; 2005b) contends that mental disorders are defined precisely to maximise prevalence. Can we conclude with Kessler that these data surprise us only because of the stigma associated with mental illness (i.e. given we all experience physical illnesses recurrently throughout our lives, why should it not be the same with mental disorders)? Should we conclude that the increase in the prevalence of mental disorders is due to the increase in stressors in our contemporary lifestyles and social changes? Should we not blur the normal/pathological boundaries if half of the population can be diagnosed with a mental disorder? Are we really becoming a *maggioranza deviante* as Basaglia (Basaglia and Ongaro Basaglia, 1971) put it, only now defined in bioeconomic rather than socioeconomic terms? Is it legitimate to include subclinical and mild disorders in prevalence, diagnostic criteria and eligibility for treatment, as Kessler seems to imply?

Although advances in biochemical research have not produced important results for psychiatric diagnosis, at least not yet, they did so as far as treatment was concerned. The hypothesis that a deficiency in serotonin could be implicated with depression led to the production and marketing of a new generation of psychiatric drugs and to the era of psychopharmacology (see Rose, 2003; 2007a; Healy, 2002). Most psychiatric drugs after chlorpromazine (tricyclics for depression, for instance) proved effective in reducing psychiatric symptoms but usually targeted several different chemical processes (see Schatzberg and Nemeroff, 2004) and their side effects were often severe. Conversely, new psychiatric drugs tend to act on very specific biochemical processes, reducing the number and severity of side effects and giving the impression if not the illusion of targeting the very specific point of origin of each single mental illness. Remarkably, Rose (2003; 2007a) has shown that this was precisely the marketing strategy of Eli Lilly when they introduced Prozac (fluoxetine hydrochloride), the first SSRI (Selective Serotonin Reuptake Inhibitor) to treat depression. The idea behind SSRIs is that once secreted, neurotransmitters are reabsorbed by the receptors to preserve them. SSRIs inhibit the reuptake process of serotonin, thus effectively increasing its levels. What is most peculiar about the new generation of psychopharmaceuticals is their *specificity* (Rose, 2007b: 149). With the advancement of biochemical research, more and more specific moods, traits and disorders are associated with specific pairs of neurotransmitters/receptors. Simultaneously, more pharmaceuticals that target those precise and specific pairs are produced, possibly reducing unwanted side effects. This reinforces all the more the 'biological dream' of psychiatry: linking mind with brain activity.

As Homer Nadesan (2008: 168) notes, psychopharmacology is, ultimately, based on the assumption that 'mental states [are] epiphenomena of brain states and that chemical imbalances in the brain produce mental imbalances'. Yet, as Healy (1997: 5) points out, advances in the study of biochemistry cannot ensure that applying a 'chemical scalpel' may prove to be the definitive answer to mental disorders,[3] because 'current understandings of brain chemistry are very incomplete and some basic tenets, such as the serotonin theory of depression, may be inaccurate' (Holmer Nadesan, 2008: 169). Several studies (e.g. Begley, 2007) point towards the view that mental states may not be an epiphenomenon of brain activity; rather, they may shape and radically change it. What is more, it is documented that the effectiveness of many psychopharmaceuticals is limited (see for instance Abboud's (2005) and Vedantam's (2006) reportages), and that in several clinical trials patients on placebos improved almost as much as those treated with the medication (e.g. Bernstein and Dooren, 2007 show that in clinical trials of SSRI antidepressants only 11 per cent of the patients on the actual drug improved more than those on the placebo).

Rose (2003) summarised the effect of such an assumption by defining the contemporary individual as a 'neurochemical self', the result of brain activity that can be enhanced, modified and restored to a 'normal' state in case an imbalance such as mental illness sets in. We understand ourselves more and more in medical terms as living beings whose lives (in the widest sense possible) are explained through the knowledge offered by the life sciences. Psychiatry is no different: we understand our states of mind in psychiatric terms, our painful experiences in terms of chemical imbalances and our processes of recovery in terms of re-establishing chemical normality.

What is more, with the ever-increasing marketing of specific molecules to target specific disorders (such as pre-menstrual syndrome, etc.) we are now witnessing a generalised reduction of mental states to brain chemistry and, at the same time, a medicalisation (psychiatrisation) of 'normal' albeit difficult and painful states of mind (such as sadness, bereavement, situational stress, etc.). From being prescribed to those suffering from a diagnosed and severe mental disorder, psychopharmaceuticals such as benzodiazepines (anxiolytics) and SSRI antidepressants are more and more used in primary-care contexts to treat minor ailments and 'subclinical' disorders such as mild insomnia, or to help people cope with difficult

---

[3] On the other hand, see the work of T.J. Crow (1980; 1986; 1990), who dedicated his research to finding an organic aetiology of schizophrenia.

phases such as bereavement or adolescence. Law (2006) has shown that pharmaceutical companies do play a role in medicalising such conditions and in shaping our understanding of mental illness.[4]

Overall, in spite of the extensive use of psychiatric drugs (be they SSRI antidepressants, antipsychotics for schizophrenia, benzodiazepines for anxiety, to cite the most used) and in spite of the evidence gathered in clinical trials, 'the modality of these drugs is mainly symptomatic', and a considerable 'proportion of users (30 to 40%) do not benefit from them' (Lehtinen et al., 2007: 140). However, psychopharmacological intervention is very cost-effective, 'compared to social-psychological interventions', and therefore appeals 'to state and private apparatuses with limited budgets' (Holmer Nadesan, 2008: 172). Rose maintains that psychopharmacology is a constitutive part of contemporary biopolitics. Psycholeptic drugs were introduced and are often still used in 'all manner of coercive situations' (Rose, 2007a: 210), a 'camicia di forza chimica' as Petrella called it (quoted in Galzigna, 2006). Nowadays, continues Rose (2007a: 210), their purpose might be rather different: their use aims to 'adjust the individual and restore and maintain his or her capacity to enter the circuits of everyday life' (especially productivity), as is the case with Bourgois's (2000) example of the use of methadone in heroin addiction rehabilitation to control unproductive individuals.

In spite of the conspicuous corpus of evidence that psychotherapeutic approaches are effective in the treatment of mental disorders, especially in conjunction with psychopharmacological intervention, they are used much less than psychopharmacology alone (Katschnig and Windhaber, 1998; Marder et al., 2003; Stiles et al., 2006). According to meta-analyses of clinical trials it has become accepted that different psychotherapeutic approaches prove effective for specific disorders. For instance, psychodynamic psychotherapies prove effective for the treatment of personality disorders and cognitive-behavioural therapy for anxiety, depression and

---

4 See also Moncrieff and Cohen (2005) for a comprehensive analysis of the assumptions that ground the 'disease-centred' model used to explain how psychopharmacology works.

bipolar disorder (Bateman and Fonagy, 2000; Roth and Fonagy, 2004; INSERM, 2004; Lehtinen et al., 2007). However, so-called 'talk therapies' are not a cost-effective intervention. Although little if any clinical evidence suggests that beyond the first year 'talk therapies' produce further improvements, psychotherapeutic approaches of any kind (from the short, problem-focused cognitive behavioural therapy to the much longer psychoanalysis) are more expensive and less readily available than psychopharmaceutical intervention, thus they are usually sought after in the private sector and by wealthier individuals. In the context of public mental health care, 'talk therapies' are rarely implemented.

Strong bilateral relationships have been established between social deprivation, exclusion, poverty and mental illness (Social Exlusion Unit, 2004). Several studies, for instance, Thornicroft (2006), show that areas of high unemployment harbour stressors and mental health problems while, at the same time, stigma, discrimination and ignorance of mental disorders often lead to a limited access to education and employment opportunities, thus to an increase of mental health problems (Sayce and Curran, 2007). Although such co-causal relationships have been documented, social interventions in psychiatry, defined as interventions that 'are not primarily directed at individual people but at the context in which they live, in order to change this context or to make it instrumental to improving symptoms and quality of life' (Lehtinen et al., 2007: 137) are rather limited. Social interventions can tackle different aspects of the problem, and can be classed according to the scale of implementation: micro-level interventions involve family and friends of the patient, meso-level interventions address the organisation and optimisation of community centres, while macro-level interventions aim at changing society and its norms as a whole (Lehtinen et al., 2007: 137) – Basaglia's struggle against the asylum and political activism would fit precisely in this last category. As a general rule, pharmacological intervention, at times paired with psychotherapeutic approaches when possible, is favoured over any form of social intervention.

One of the key mental health recommendations of WHO has been to move mental health care from an institutionalised setting (such as the psychiatric hospital) to community and primary care (WHO, 2011: 9). Data collected in the WHO *Mental Health Atlas* in 2011 seems reassuring, in that it indicates that mental hospital beds are decreasing in the majority of countries (WHO, 2011: 9). However, the paradigm of deinstitutionalisation – which consists of moving mental health care away from institutional contexts such as the psychiatric hospital into community and small-scale clinics, and empowering outpatients, for instance involving them in treatment decisions – is still being implemented very slowly on a global scale. Only 44 per cent of countries have a majority of facilities that provide psychosocial intervention and, while 77 per cent of individuals admitted to a mental hospital remain inpatients for less than a year, almost a quarter of hospitalisations are still longer (WHO, 2011: 11). Unsurprisingly, higher-income countries have fifty-eight times more outpatient mental health facilities than low-income ones (WHO, 2011: 10). Of the countries that have moved most of their mental health care from the hospital to the community centres, many are witnessing a phase that has been termed 'reinstitutionalisation', as many of the former inpatients are now treated in alternative residential facilities, prisons or even criminal psychiatric hospitals or secure forensic units (Priebe et al., 2005). In those countries that have yet to broadly implement deinstitutionalisation (for instance, the former Eastern bloc countries in Europe, see Tomov et al., 2007), numerous abuses of human rights still occur and patient empowerment and community care are very far from being put into practice (Mental Disability Advocacy Center, 2005; Knapp et al., 2007: 4).

Overall, if we were to draw a line and briefly assess the state of psychiatry at the time of writing it could be said that approaches and efficacy differ greatly from country to country but that general trends can be identified. There is a general consensus that the aetiology and pathogenesis of 'functional' (non-organic) mental disorders (i.e. the majority of mental illnesses) are biopsychosocial, although the boundaries and contributions of the biological, psychological and social dimensions are yet to be agreed upon. However, clinical practice differs substantially from this assessment. Diagnosis is purely symptomatic and treatment is at least predominantly pharmaceutical, with some psychotherapeutic support, especially in the private sector, and very limited social interventions.

Governamentality, Biopolitics and Psychiatry

Thus far, I have presented an overview of psychiatry as it is currently practised at a 'micro-level'; that is, in a clinical setting. However, we have seen, thanks to Foucault's work among others, that at a certain point in history psychiatry – and medicine in general – begins to be involved with society at a macro-level. In the first place, it is a matter of judiciary measures and expertise: psychiatrists are called to assess the intentionality of crimes, and the mental health of criminals, to judge whether they could plead extenuating circumstances. This makes psychiatry into a science of abnormality in general, not only in a criminal context: psychiatrists begin to assess patterns of abnormality in the population, to look for the signs of a possible future abnormality, in order to prevent the alleged danger that a full-blown derangement could entail.

In the context of the biopolitical rationalisation of the art of governance that Foucault described, psychiatry has also somewhat shifted its line of intervention, especially at the macro-level. First and foremost, it must be noted that psychiatry has become more and more the medicine of mental health rather than the medicine of mental disorder. Along with most other branches of physical medicine, psychiatry has become a science of promoting and maintaining 'good health', mental health in this case.

According to Rose (2001: 27), this should be understood in the light of a recent shift within biopolitics, which he terms 'ethopolitics': 'if discipline individualizes and normalizes, and biopower collectivizes and socializes, ethopolitics concerns itself with the self-techniques by which human beings should judge themselves and act upon themselves to make themselves better than they are'. Under this definition, Rose collates numerous aspects that have contributed to an internal shift in biopolitics. While, in Foucault's first definition, the object of biopolitics was the population and its purpose was the well-being of the nation, now biopolitics returns to focus on the individual, no longer simply managing it statistically, as part of a population. Ethopolitics encourages individuals to embark on a quest for well-being, for instance by inducing them to use the gym more often, to follow a more balanced dietary regime, to become more aware of self-medication, and so on. This intervention is extremely cost-effective, especially in those countries with a public health care system, in that by making individuals introject a certain ideal of health and thus regulating their daily routines, the cost of medical intervention is effectively cut: more 'balanced' lifestyles reduce the risk of cancer, a better diet reduces obesity and obesity-related conditions, etc.

Like disciplinary power, which, according to Foucault, produced the modern individual, ethopolitics, according to Rose, creates a 'somatic self', in that we understand ourselves more and more in somatic terms. At the same time, political and especially ethical praxis 'increasingly take[s] the body as the key site for work on the self' (Rose, 2001: 17). In psychiatry, such an ethopolitical regime is evident in a number of paradigm shifts, which Rose also notes, such as Kramer's (1993) famous notion of 'cosmetic psychopharmacology', the use of psychopharmaceuticals to enhance, boost or otherwise optimise and maximise mental, cognitive and behavioural functions. Cosmetic psychopharmacology could be regarded as an extreme pole of the 'consumerisation' and commercialisation of psychiatry. However, with the increasing medicalisation and psychiatrisation of normal, albeit painful, states, such as bereavement, situational stress, and so on, the campaigns for the optimisation of mental health (such as Gibson's 'five-a-day for the mind'[5]) are indeed becoming more and more evident, an overarching tendency that Tarizzo (2011) calls the 'behavioural optimisation of the populational man'.

Yet, as we have seen, biopolitics does not only act in the direction of optimisation and maximisation of life; it also acts somehow 'negatively', in a preventive and limiting way. With this in mind, Braun (2007: 23) contends that, if we ask ourselves in which modalities does biological existence concern politics, we cannot answer exclusively with Rose's ethopolitics. We need to analyse a second and possibly more important aspect, that of 'biosecurity':

> If security is a political discourse that justifies new forms of sovereign power by placing the actions of the state 'outside' politics, then biosecurity risks doing much the same, justifying a continuous state of emergency at the level of political life by reference to a

---

5 See <http://www.mindapple.org>, accessed 10 June 2012.

> continuous state of emergence at the level of molecular life. We might conclude, then, that biosecurity names much more than a set of political technologies whose purpose is to govern the disorder of biological life; it increasingly names a global project that seeks to achieve certain biomolecular futures by pre-empting others, and does so in part by reconfiguring in other places relations between people, and between people and their animals. Biosecurity weds biopolitics with geopolitics. (Braun, 2007: 23)

While ethopolitics creates new forms of pastoral power – to foster, optimise and manage biological life – the net of biosecurity has, according to Braun, justified a resurgence of sovereign power, in the name of preventing the spread of contaminants, illnesses and pollution. While the body that Rose describes is a governed body, subject to the introjection of ethical practices that seek to maximise and optimise it, the body Braun describes is 'embedded in a chaotic and unpredictable molecular world, a body understood in terms of a general economy of exchange and circulation, haunted by the spectre of newly emerging or still unspecifiable risks' (Braun, 2007: 14). More than being concerned about the 'care for the self', governing such a vulnerable and fragile body – immersed in what Vallat (quoted in Braun, 2007: 8) called the 'great biological cauldron', constantly exposed to pandemic viruses, hygienic risks, natural catastrophes, environmental pollution, stressors of all sorts – is a matter of managing 'imminent catastrophe' (Braun, 2007: 8).

The notion of biosecurity fits perfectly with psychiatry: as we have seen, according to epidemiological studies, most people have suffered or will suffer from a mental disorder in their lifetime, therefore the risk of mental illness is embedded in the population and in our very lifestyle, full of possible stressors and traumatic experiences. One of the most influential models of mental health, which expands on Engel's biopsychosocial one, is Zubin and Spring's (1977) stress-vulnerability model, according to which each individual has different strengths and vulnerabilities, considered from biological, psychological and social perspectives. The lower the vulnerability in one of the three aspects, the higher the amount of stress the individual can withstand before a mental disorder develops. Managing such risk factors is among the top priorities of policy-makers in the context of mental health care, and WHO recommendations highlight the centrality of promoting mental health to prevent the onset of mental disorders. Such promotion should be capillary and focus, first and foremost, on introducing psychiatric consultations and screenings in primary health care (GPs and so on). Among other suggestions we could include, for instance,

> parent training programmes and interventions for the early identification of mental health problems in schools, flexible practices and access to counselling and support in the workplace, and bereavement counselling and social activities to reduce isolation and the risk of depression in older age. (Knapp et al., 2007: 11)

Some studies (Kazdin, 1996; Schoevers et al., 2006) indeed suggest that symptoms such as mild depression might be partially prevented with intervention in early life. However, there is very little further evidence that psychiatry can prevent mental disorders at all (Paris, 2008: 194).

Overall, psychiatry, medicine and epidemiology, among other disciplines and sciences that run parallel to biopolitics, ethopolitics and biosecurity, allow 'new forms of subjectivity' to emerge (Meloni, 2011: 157). As Rose highlights, we come to know ourselves more and more in somatic terms, for instance, understanding our traits as inherited genetic material or avoiding risk factors through diets and fitness programmes. Rose extends such understanding to the mind by coining the idea of 'neurochemical selves': the more research advances, the more we understand not only our existence but our mental processes, behaviours, moods and feelings in terms of neurotransmitters, neural and brain activity. *Vis-à-vis* this biological reductionism, which flattens psychosocial life on biological life, there is the whole structure of governamentality, understood both in terms of ethopolitics – that is to say, the introjection of affirmative and optimising conducts – and of biosecurity – the prevention of illnesses and disorders. This structure contributes to the creation of individuals who, on the one hand, aim at 'biological perfection' (at times even medically enhanced), while, on the other, perceive themselves as thrown into the menacing 'biological cauldron' full of contaminants and pollutants, always at risk, intrinsically fragile and mortal.

Psychiatry, in a biopolitical context, is, simply put, the biological medicine of mental health. Its main aim seems to be to reduce psychological suffering, in all its forms, by applying the most holistic of approaches, based on a biopsychosocial model. *De facto*, however, psychiatry contributes to the emergence of a fragile subjectivity, always in need of preventive measures, support and endorsement, and to the levelling of the psychosocial into the biological: it medicalises painful albeit normal states, it offers the 'dream' of a cosmetic psychopharmacology, ready to optimise and maximise psychosocial and cognitive functions, it promises the containment and prevention of mental disorders, the increase of mental well-being.

The Second Biological Psychiatry, Biopolitics and Italy

Such considerations provide an overview of psychiatry as it is generally practised in western countries and of the concerns that it raises among critics. In Italy the situation, mostly due to Law 180 and the successful closure of psychiatric hospitals, is comparable albeit slightly different. Taking into account the limited number of studies and surveys conducted on mental health care in Italy, the first key aspect to consider is the number of inpatient beds available. Due to the closure of psychiatric hospitals, since 1978 there has been a steady decline in residential inpatient facilities and beds offered, amounting to a striking 85.9 per cent in 2000 (Rose, 2007b). In 2009, according to the WHO's 'European Health for All database' (WHO, 2012), Italy counted 10.59 inpatient beds per 100,000 population, the lowest in the world. Such inpatient beds are located in public general hospital psychiatric units (the *Servizio Psichiatrico di Diagnosi e Cura*, with a maximum of fifteen beds each). However, since the reform, the number of private inpatient beds has remained stable and the latest data available (the PROGRES study conducted by De Girolamo and others)[6] has shown that, in the year 2000 there were 1,374 private residential facilities offering 17,343 inpatient beds (although the numbers remain low in comparison to the rest of Europe, this data means that inpatient residential facilities in the private sector outnumber those in the public sector by three to one). The type and quality of treatment offered in these facilities is very difficult

---

6 Gruppo Nazionale PROGRES, 2001; Picardi et al., 2003.

to monitor, in part because of a lack of surveys and also because Italy does not have an accreditation system (De Girolamo et. al., 2007). Outpatient community services are offered by 707 *Centri di Salute Mentale*, 612 day centres (WHO, 2005: 251–52), 1,107 clinics and 309 day hospitals (Maone et al., 2002).

Overall, from this data it can be said, following De Girolamo et al. (2007: 89), that deinstitutionalisation in Italy has been by and large successful, albeit unevenly across different regions. By comparison, it is interesting to note that crimes committed by mental outpatients have not increased during the process of deinstitutionalisation (Priebe et al., 2005). More interesting still is the fact, noted by Rose (2007b), that, although the number of available inpatient beds has drastically decreased in comparison to other European countries, comparatively, the use of psychopharmaceuticals has not increased dramatically. From 1993 to 2002 the use of antidepressants and mood stabilisers almost doubled (6,727 to 11,155 SUs per 1,000 population), that of antipsychotics and anxiolytics has slightly increased (4,292 to 5,558 for antipsychotic and 22,549 to 23,416 for anxiolytics), while psychostimulants (mainly amphetamines used to treat attention deficit hyperactivity disorder, ADHD), have never been used. In spite of the increase, the prescribing of psychopharmaceuticals is among the lowest in Europe, except for anxiolytics, which is average (Rose, 2007b).

If, comparatively, the use of psychopharmaceuticals is below average, it is still rather high and has indeed grown through recent decades, which was foreseeable. Psychosocial interventions, in spite of the widespread community approach, have not achieved a diffusion comparable to pharmaceutical interventions (Morlino et al., 1993; Magliano et al., 2002). What is more, as De Girolamo et al. (2007: 87) note in summarising a number of surveys (Barbui et al., 1999; Munizza et al., 1995; Tibaldi et al., 1997; Tognoni, 1999; Tomasi et al., 2006), in Italy, as often as in other countries (Harrington et al., 2002; Paris, 2008), co-morbid diagnoses and the consequent use of poly-pharmacy are common. Prescription patterns are often inconsistent and 'at odds with current guidelines and recommendations' (De Girolamo, 2007: 87) and, as Piccione (2004: 14) stresses, only 15 per cent of administered therapies are backed by evidence-based medicine and clinical trials.

This data does not allow for any definitive assessment of mental health care in Italy. Tentatively, it could be said that the general trend of the 'second biological psychiatry' as Shorter called it, is spreading also in Italy, although at a different pace and to a different extent when compared to other countries. Certainly, the coercive component of the old psychiatry, with its involuntary treatments and often lifelong admission to the asylum is, generally speaking, over, although at times scattered reports of physical restraint and abysmal treatments in specific *Centri di Salute Mentale* and *Servizi Psichiatrici di Diagnosi e Cura* do surface.[7] The link between justice and psychiatry that raised so many concerns, most notably Foucault's, seems to be in the process of being undone, as, following Senator Ignazio Marino's inspection in 2011, the six last remaining criminal psychiatric hospitals (*OPG, Ospedale Psichiatrico Giudiziario*), will close by 2013.

However, in spite of the comparatively broader community approach, and the successes of deinstitutionalisation, Italian psychiatry is still subject to harsh criticism by psychiatrists of the 'Basaglian' legacy, such as Dell'Acqua, who recently (2008a) criticised extensively the widespread and inconsistent use of psychopharmacology in Italy. In his recent assessment of Italian psychiatric health care, Colucci worriedly presents a scenario that also confirms the rise of the 'second biological psychiatry' in Italy. While Franco Rotelli (2005: 39) had already anticipated that 'oggi il campo è [...] dominato in Italia e ovunque [dalle] forme di surmedicalizzazione della follia', Colucci (2008: 118) adds that there are hardly any practices of 'assistenza e [...] presa in carico della persona sul territorio, nella comunità', and psychiatric assistance is mostly confined to arranging

---

7   See, for instance, the anonymous report on Viareggio, at http://www.news-forumsa-lutementale.it/viareggio-buone-o-cattive-pratiche/ [accessed 10 June 2012], Franco Mastrogiovanni's case (http://www.agoravox.it/Francesco-Mastrogiovanni-morte.html [accessed 10 June 2012]), cases of physical coercion in the *Dipartimento di Salute Mentale* in Enna (http://www.vivienna.it/2011/02/20/enna-malasanita-in-psichiatria/ [accessed 10 June 2012]), the seven controversial deaths in Milan's Niguarda hospital (http://affaritaliani.libero.it/sociale/morti_reparti_psichiatrici_ospedale_niguarda_milano220311.html?refresh_ce [accessed 10 June 2012]) or Bo's (2012) report on Mantova's *Servizio Psichiatrico di Diagnosi e Cura*.

for the patient's admission into a public hospital.[8] The medicalisation of psychiatry is advocated as a necessary step, 'dopo anni di "oscurantismo" e "ignoranza"' towards the 'riconversione della psichiatria in disciplina scientifica' (Colucci, 2008: 121). Likewise, Di Vittorio (2006: 75) observes that, after Basaglia, Italian psychiatry 'fails to understand how the "good" mental health policy [...] can easily become the best alibi for a "bad" mental health policy', a policy that

> involves control and social normalization through an apparatus of generalized prevention of pathology risks and the massive prescription of psycholeptic drugs. (Di Vittorio, 2006: 75)

Basaglia was well aware he was witnessing the beginning of such an era; however, he was not able to develop this observation much further. He acknowledged that Law 180 was not a 'panacea a tutti i problemi del malato mentale', because it eventually encouraged 'omologare la psichiatria alla medicina, cioè il comportamento umano al corpo [anatomico]', which Basaglia deemed as paradoxical as 'omologare i cani con le banane' (Basaglia, 1978a: 11). During a conference in Belo Horizonte on 17 November 1979, less than a year before his death, he stressed that the asylum was no longer 'nelle mura'. On the contrary, it is in our everyday lives, because we are 'medicalizzati e psichiatrizzati ogni volta che andiamo dal medico' (Basaglia, 2000: 176). Basaglia (2000: 181) is clear on this point: 'su questo nuovo manicomio dobbiamo agire'. In the 'ideological gap' that the reform created, Basaglia (2000: 189) witnessed a 'ridefinizione in termini territoriali della logica manicomiale'. As he feared, instead of being allowed to move forward from the ideological gap left by the reform, psychiatrists were required to produce an alternative to disciplinary psychiatry. As Foucault remarked, notably in agreement with Basaglia's position,

---

8 The Italian National Statistical Institute (*ISTAT*) has published a detailed analysis of the hospitalisation of patients suffering from a psychiatric disorder in the years 1999–2004. This data confirms Colucci's claim. The *Nota Informativa* of 2008 states that most admissions, 99.6 per cent, take place in public or private hospitals. Of these 92.7 per cent are acute disorders, 3.1 per cent are chronic disorders and 4.2 per cent are rehab (ISTAT, 2008: 3).

as soon as one proposes, one proposes a vocabulary, an ideology, which can only have effects of domination. What we have to present are instruments and tools that people might find useful. (Cooper et al., 1988: 197)

Law 180 was only a part, albeit radical and revolutionary, of a process of transformation for psychiatry that, for good or for ill, brought mental health care to the state I have described so far. Basaglia witnessed only the beginning of this and he seemed somewhat critical of this development. We must however bear in mind that much has changed since his early, tentative criticism, and there is a general consensus that the advances in psychiatry brought about many improvements in the quality of life of those who suffer from a mental disorder, and of their families. Severe psychotic symptoms can not only be kept at bay but also reduced without physical constraint and without debilitating side effects, long-term internment is no longer advocated as a necessary measure, social and economic conditions are better monitored to prevent the onset of ensuing mental disorders. Basaglia always conceded that psychopharmacological intervention was an effective treatment to mental illness, which he regarded as real and biological, as much as flu or cancer. Yet, he also always argued against reducing mental illness to being *simply* an organic condition, urging psychiatrists to embrace a biopsychosocial perspective, thus differentiating the therapeutic approaches and adopting a holistic perspective (understood as taking into account all aspects of the person, not as the alternative medicine that has recently taken shape) that would not ignore the social conditions of those suffering from a mental disorder in favour of their organic bodies or psychological and cognitive functions. As a matter of fact, although Basaglia never seemed to prescribe precise guidelines on how to carry out deinstitutionalisation nor on how to practise psychiatry, towards the end of his life, during a conference in Brazil, he urged psychiatrists to (2000: 167) 'trovare un contenuto reale di questa [...] psichiatria alternativa', the grounds on which to affirmatively build a practice beyond the denial of institutional psychiatry and the refusal of the role of traditional psychiatrists. The asylum could only be dismantled but psychiatry had to be reformed, not erased.

I strongly agree with Colucci, who, very aptly, summarised Basaglia's proposal for an alternative psychiatry as 'una clinica del soggetto attraverso la cura dei suoi legami sociali e la ricostruzione della sua appartenenza a una *polis*' (Colucci, 2008: 115): a definition that accounts for the biopsychosocial model and gives a clear idea of a possible holistic approach in psychiatry. However, this definition can be applied seamlessly in the context of Basaglia's early career, when the struggle against the 'total institution' of the asylum justified the need for a strong definition of subjectivity, a notion to oppose the objectification of the first biological reductionism of early institutional psychiatry, and *polis* could be easily regarded as the 'outside', the place from which the mentally ill person was excluded, and in which reintegration could prove as controversial as exclusion. In an advanced state of biopolitics, such definitions are more difficult to shape consistently and, with a widespread psychiatrisation of everyday life and normal states, with the looming issue of biosecurity that monitors and screens the population to maximise mental health from childhood, with a constant promotion of mental as much as physical well-being, along with the economic advantages that such well-being carries, the attempt to define a 'subjectivity' and a *polis* rebuilt around the subject proves much more controversial.

In the concluding chapter of this book I begin to untangle this knot and try to read Basaglia's work through the lens of biopolitics. In a biopolitical state of affairs, what is a 'subject'? Is there a *polis* where the (psychotic) subject belongs? What is the contribution of psychiatry towards the definition of the subject, the *polis* and the act of belonging to a *polis*? Has Basaglia's legacy been betrayed by the rise of a 'biopolitical psychiatry', as many critics seem to suggest, or can we find a positive continuity? And, all things considered, are biopolitics and psychiatry in a biopolitical state as negative, coercive and controlling as many critics seem to believe?

Of course, from a certain point of view, when cognitive, behavioural and psychological activity are flattened into brain, neuronal and ultimately chemical activity, we can easily see how the biopsychosocial model is eventually reduced to a biological model. Not only are psychological and social features overlooked in favour of 'biological' ones, but, further, the diversity and individuality of each person is lost, insofar as we can all be 'reduced' to our shared organic traits. We can be understood as the 'human species', whose neurotransmitters work in the same way in every single individual and whose psychological differences are mere surface epiphenomena of comparable chemistry. Similarly, the social, collective and community aspect is levelled onto the 'populational': although Rose has shown that new forms of socialisation are born of biological reductionism (for instance, 'biological citizenship' in Rose and Novas, 2004), we can see how the collective aspect that most interests psychiatrists and policy-makers might be the populational, statistical, the normalised model of the human being, where disorders are understood in epidemiological terms of prevalence and not as symptoms of an individual suffering. If, on the one hand, the subject is flattened onto its own somatic entity, the group of subjects, the community, is flattened onto the population, the epidemiologically relevant collective. Nevertheless, there might be more to biopolitics and biopolitical psychiatry: if most critics tend to show their negative, coercive, reductive and destructive aspects, there are also possible affirmative and positive outcomes that might even be retrieved from Basaglia's work.

CHAPTER 6

Towards an Affirmative Biopolitical Psychiatry

Introduction

Two central notions characterise Basaglia's work and his utopian vision: 'subject' and 'community'. It is on these that I wish to focus in this final chapter of the book. Before we consider whether a 'contenuto reale' for alternative psychiatry (Basaglia, 2000: 167) can indeed be found in the 'libretto rosso' that was metaphorically waved in protest, the 'libretto rosso' has to be reread in the light of biopolitics, so as to show that its revolutionary potential has indeed not been quashed by the rise of a 'politics of life', as some critics seem to imply. Its revolutionary potential should be sought in its capacity to continuously engender a new praxis – or, better still, *praxes* – that do not 'crystallise' in set and 'effective' responses to inconvenient problems such as deviance or the pathogenic potential of social norms. Basaglia attributed the capacity to continuously engender new praxes that better respond to the needs of the people to the idea of utopia, which he regarded as the 'elemento prefigurante' that prevents reality from falling into stasis. I believe the 'elementi prefiguranti' that allow us to read Basaglia in the age of biopolitics are in fact two ontologies: that of the 'subject' and that of the 'community'.

This chapter, therefore, begins by presenting the ontology of the subject as it is found in Basaglia's work, in comparison to Foucault's. I then discuss the notion of 'community' in relation to that of 'population' and, finally, I articulate Basaglia's conceptualisation of communitarian relationship in conjunction with his idea of subjectivity and Esposito's notions of *communitas* and *immunitas*. The purpose of this analysis is to outline an affirmative biopolitics or, at least, an affirmative biopolitical psychiatry, as found in Basaglia's utopian work.

La clinica del soggetto: Subjectivity and Individuality

The point of departure for Basaglia's criticism of institutional psychiatry, which led him to envision Law 180 and the dismantling of the asylum, was, arguably, the centrality of the patient's subjectivity, as opposed to the 'objectification' that institutionalisation and biological reductionism carried out. In spite of his increased attention towards social norms, political activism, and so forth, the centrality Basaglia ascribed to the notion of subject remains unaltered throughout his struggle against the asylum. At the centre of his struggle there is always the former inpatient, the person who is suffering from a mental disorder. To this extent, Colucci indeed grasped the essence of Basaglia's proposal in defining it as a 'clinica del soggetto'. However, as I show in this section, thanks to the work of Foucault, among others, the notion of subjectivity becomes rather controversial, and must be at least disambiguated before we embrace the notion that Basaglia's clinical approach can indeed be regarded as a 'clinica del soggetto'.

According to Foucault, the individual, being always-already woven into countless power relations, is an effect of power itself. This is clear, for instance, in *Psychiatric Power*, where Foucault (2006b: 56) suggests that the individual is nothing but the result of certain 'techniques of political power', such as 'uninterrupted supervision, continual writing and potential punishment'. Also, the process of individualisation entails several other techniques which he describes elsewhere: examination (Foucault, 1991: 184–92), expertise (2003a: 1–30), normalisation (1991: 182–83), and so on. Up to this point, Foucault is referring to the individual, with little mention of the notion of subject. In his later works, when the concept of subject becomes central, it is never completely clear whether or not Foucault regards the subject as something different from the individual. It could be suggested that, while the individual is the effect of power as regards social relations, the subject is the effect of power as regards the reflexive relation. That is to say, one is under an effect of power when one is in a relationship with others (individuality) but is under the same effect also when one is alone with oneself (subjectivity). I will return to this point shortly.

A clarifying statement towards a definition of the Foucauldian subject can be found in 'The Subject and Power', the afterword that Foucault contributed to Dreyfus and Rabinow's *Michel Foucault: Beyond Structuralism and Hermeneutics*. As Foucault (1982: 208) says, his objective throughout his work 'has been to create a history of the different modes by which human beings are made subjects'. Arguably, he is implying by this statement that human beings are not of themselves subjects but are *made* so. The very noun 'subject' suggests an ambiguity: subject means both who/what performs the action expressed by the verb and he/she who is subject to power; for instance, the subject of a sovereign. Hence, we can assume that, according to Foucault, individuality is not a state of subjection to social norms that is logically and ontogenetically preceded by subjectivity: there is no 'free' subject that pre-exists social norms and political power and that then, at a second stage, somehow 'alienates' into a notion of individuality. Subjectivity in itself is always-already a state of subjection to power. This conclusion is endorsed in *Hermeneutics of the Subject* (Foucault, 2005), where Foucault (1982: 208) goes so far as to maintain that not only are human beings *made* into subjects, they also turn themselves into subjects through a number of techniques such as the examination of conscience or spiritual exercises. Subjectivity in itself is the product of several 'technologies of the self' (Foucault, 1988), which

> permit individuals to effect by their own means [...] a certain number of operations on their own bodies and souls, thoughts, conduct, and way of being, so as to transform themselves in order to attain a certain state of happiness, purity, wisdom, perfection, or immortality. (Foucault, 1988: 18)

Through these technologies, individuals become capable of self-discipline and self-control. Not even the Socratic 'know yourself' (Foucault, 1997b: 28) can be regarded as independent from relations of power. For instance, we have seen how, according to Rose, our self-understanding is shaped by medical and psychopharmacological concepts – he summarises it through the notion of 'somatic' and 'neurochemical selves' – or, again, with reference to the social sciences and psychology, how 'one comes to know oneself [...] in relation to behavioural, cognitive, and emotional norms generated by the social sciences' (Holmer Nadesan, 2008: 153).

What matters for Foucault is that, ultimately, there is no need for someone to wield power, because subjects are themselves a product of self-disciplining techniques and are thus always under a permanent effect of power. This was already clear to Foucault in *Discipline and Punish*, where he suggests that the ultimate aim of panopticism was precisely to create a surveillance that is 'permanent in its effects, even if it is discontinuous in its action' (Foucault, 1991: 201). Inmates do not know when the supervisor is actually inside the central tower of the *Panopticon*, so they constantly believe that they might be under surveillance. Eventually, they are 'caught up in a power situation of which they are themselves the bearers' (Foucault, 1991: 201). Power no longer emanates from a centre, such as the sovereign or the supervisor; it is the subjects who exert power over themselves: instead of 'il dominio sull'oggetto', the generalisation of panopticism inaugurates 'la [...] partecipazione soggettiva [dell'oggetto] all'atto della dominazione' (Esposito, 2004: 29).

This is why, according to Rovatti (2008: 217), '[il] soggetto [...], per Foucault, non c'è, è un'invenzione piena di conseguenze negative e perfino distruttive'. The very notion of subjectivity is the mark of one's alienation and loss of freedom. The negative consequences of clinging to a substantive notion of subjectivity amount to the fact that,

> mentre noi crediamo di segnare, attraverso la singolarità delle nostre esperienze interne ed esterne, un territorio individuale, [...] libero, in realtà ci chiudiamo [...] nella prigione della nostra soggettività individuale [...] e ci rendiamo docili [e] agenti di questo potere. (Rovatti, 2008: 224)

In short, borrowing Seigel's words (1990: 276), 'sought in the name of freedom, such subjectivity opened individuals to domination by the powers'. There is no such thing as an independent subject, as the very way we perceive ourselves is already determined by relations of power.

The tension between subjectivity and individuality and their being always-already woven into relations of power, points to a wider ambiguity in Foucault's *oeuvre*: that between the '*tecniche politiche* con le quali lo Stato assume e integra al suo interno la cura della vita naturale degli individui' and the

> *tecnologie del sé*, attraverso le quali si attua il processo di soggettivazione che porta l'individuo a vincolarsi alla propria identità e alla propria coscienza e, insieme, a un potere di controllo esterno. (Agamben, 2005: 8)

While, arguably, the production of individuals through political techniques and the production of subjects through the technologies of the self are interconnected, 'il punto in cui questi due aspetti del potere convergono è rimasto, tuttavia, singolarmente in ombra nella ricerca di Foucault' (Agamben, 2005: 8). At the same time, the distinction between individuality and subjectivity has remained blurred. Although Foucault never clearly advances a complete convergence of individuality and subjectivity, from his writings it is not always clear if it is possible to trace a clear-cut distinction between the two notions or if a subject is, all things considered, an individual. It seems to me that Foucault very often implies that human beings are always-already subjects (i.e. subject to self-disciplining techniques) *and* individuals (i.e. individuated and individualised by a network of power relations). Although we can theoretically distinguish between subjectivity and individuality in order to distinguish between the effects of self-disciplining techniques and the effects of social relations of power, there is no such thing as a subject who is not an individual.

Subjectivity, to Foucault, is therefore as misleading a notion as individuality: the more one deludes oneself into believing one is conquering a 'subjective' and 'individual' dimension, the more one weaves oneself into power relations. In Basaglia, we encounter a similar albeit subtly different and somehow more 'optimistic' conceptualisation of subjectivity. Before discussing Basaglia's notion of subject, it is important to remember that he can be imprecise in his use of words. In his early works, it is quite clear that when he mentions the terms 'soggetto' and 'soggettività' he is using them in a phenomenological/existentialist way, in opposition to the traditional medical conception of the subject/object relationship. After the 'political turn' in 1964, his language becomes less specific. He often uses the terms *soggetto*, *individuo* and also *persona* interchangeably. Yet, despite the fact that Basaglia never developed a precise and explicit definition of subjectivity, it is possible to outline his notion of the subject, or, at least, of the 'enigma della soggettività in psichiatria' (1965a), from the conclusions drawn in the earlier chapters.

As noted already in Chapter 2, in *Corpo e istituzione* (1967), Basaglia refers to an Oriental tale which tells of a snake that entered a man through his mouth and from there controlled him for a long time: this is the 'condizione istituzionale del malato mentale'. Through this tale, Basaglia (1967a: 106) wants to exemplify the 'incorporazione da parte del malato di un nemico che lo distrugge'. This is not only the condition of the inmate in the old asylum but also a risk for social and community approaches in psychiatry – based on the chimaera of rehabilitation: 'le nuove tecniche su cui si fonda la riabilitazione [...] vengono esportate come nuovo mezzo di manipolazione delle masse' (Basaglia, 1971b: 207–8). Basaglia is here stressing that human beings are indeed so much woven into power relations that power is no longer exerted from above but also from within. Although this brings Basaglia and Foucault very close to one another, it must be noted that, to Basaglia, the subject is not *only* an effect of power.

In his early thought Basaglia refers to the subject using a Heideggerian-Binswangerian vocabulary: subjectivity corresponds to the *Dasein*, to the being-in-the-world, the intrinsic capacity of creating projects for one's life: in short, 'il soggetto esiste solo nella misura nella quale "è" al mondo' (Basaglia, 1953a: 5). This should already suggest that, if there is such a thing as a 'Basaglian subject', it cannot be regarded as something substantial – 'con tutte le sue più irrinunziabili connotazioni metafisiche di unità, assolutezza, interiorità' (Esposito, 1998: 10) – first and foremost, because, as I have discussed earlier, the most important characteristic of the subject is its inability to establish a direct reflexive relationship without the existence of the other. The subject, according to Basaglia, is constitutionally woven into intersubjectivity: the subject cannot perceive itself as such, as an individual subject, different from all other subjects, without accepting the unavoidability of a negotiated relationship with the other. Although a gap must be established between the subject and the other – a distance, a space for subjectification – it is thanks to the objectifying presence of the other that one becomes and is a subject. Without a world to which one can relate there is no subjectivity.

This can be regarded as a constitutional, constitutive and even somehow paradoxical *lack* in subjectivity: the more one withdraws from the other, attempting to establish an insurmountable distance in order to safeguard one's individual subjectivity, to defend it against the determining influence of the other, the more one loses sight of one's being a subject, and thus 'fades', engendering, for instance, symptoms such as derealisation and depersonalisation. This is what Basaglia summarises as the tension between *alienità* and *alterità*: the less one accepts one's *alterità* the more one falls into a state of *alienità*. This is also the core notion of what Basaglia, borrowing Husserl's expression (1970: 5), refers to as the 'enigma della soggettività in psichiatria', which I would summarise as the 'constitutional lack of the subject': intersubjectivity logically and ontogenetically precedes subjectivity and it is only by participating in intersubjectivity while not losing oneself in it that one becomes a subject. There is no subject outside of intersubjectivity.

This is why the 'Basaglian' subject cannot be regarded as 'substantial'. Rather, I would suggest regarding it as a utopian construction. In Chapter 4, I showed how, according to Basaglia (1975a: 254), utopias are those ideas that help to shape reality; they may be goals that are unattainable but any practice that aspires to change a crystallised *status quo* must nevertheless regard them as a guide. Utopias should foreshadow reality as they are a constant search to meet the needs of the people, says Basaglia. Reality should be constantly shaped and reshaped in terms of utopian aims and is thus an unstable condition, open to being shaped according to the needs of people. Utopias are what prevents reality from becoming static; that is to say – in Foucault's and Basaglia's terms – 'crystallised' into a state of domination.

In the specific case of the alternative psychiatry Basaglia advocates, it seems to me that subjectivity plays the part of one of the two fundamental utopian constructions that should guide everyday practice. Even if the subject, strictly speaking in Foucauldian terms, does not exist, and even if it is an effect of power relations, somehow 'returning' to it in psychiatry – that is, overcoming medical objectification, disregarding reductive clinical categories, etc. – does have counter-hegemonic effects, it does provide an effective form of resistance. The subject to which a return is advocated is neither substantial, nor solipsistic, nor does it transcend intersubjectivity

– Basaglia would not propose to reintroduce a somehow spiritual dimension to psychiatry: it is a constitutionally lacking subject, continuously exposed to taxing and determining relations of power – which are imposed both from above and from within the subject. Necessarily, the notion of subjectivity that is recuperated in this way is not isolated: the constitutional lack of the subject entails that the very nature of subjectivity is to be in constant and radical need of the other.

It may be that there is no real 'way out' of a Foucauldian notion of individual/subject, being, as it is, the effect of power relations; it may be that it is not possible to 'svuotare [il soggetto], liberar[lo] da se stesso' (Rovatti, 2008: 219); nonetheless, psychiatry should always aim to 'restituir[e] la soggettività' (Colucci, 1995: 92) to the mentally sick person. According to Basaglia, whilst the *individual* may be the effect *of* power relations, a psychiatrist should assume that the *subject* cannot be reduced *to* such power relations. Through strategies of resistance such as the struggle of local intellectuals or the 'bracketing' of mental illness it seems to be somehow possible to recover a hypothetical and paradoxical – Basaglia would say enigmatic – subjectivity, maybe one innocent of the effect of power relations, even if this amounts only to a constitutional lack, the radical need of the other.

Nevertheless, disambiguating the notion of subject as one of the possible ontological foundations of Basaglia's clinical approach does not automatically disambiguate the whole notion of a 'clinica del soggetto'. Why should a clinical approach based on such a notion of subjectivity not reintroduce patients into an alienating society, thus reproducing the risks of social psychiatry, for instance? How can a 'cura dei legami sociali', which Colucci likens to the 'clinica del soggetto', be grounded on different premises compared to a rehabilitative social and community psychiatry? Are they not suspiciously similar? All things considered, why should the utopian notion of a 'constitutional lack of the subject' encourage a less coercive and objectifying psychiatry? To try to clarify these doubts, I believe a second utopian construction must be introduced: Basaglia's notion of community.

La cura dei legami sociali: Community and Population

Colucci's definition of Basaglia's clinical approach can be divided into two parts: 'clinica del soggetto' and 'cura dei suoi legami sociali e [...] ricostruzione della sua appartenenza a una *polis*' (Colucci, 2008: 115). I have partially disambiguated the first part: if the subject is constitutionally lacking then a clinic of the subject should not be regarded as a therapeutic approach aimed at strengthening subjectivity or individuality but at re-establishing and renegotiating the logical and ontogenetic primacy of intersubjectivity. To this extent, re-establishing the social bonds and rebuilding the sense of belonging to the *polis* is parallel to the clinic of the subject, in that the very 'core' of subjectivity is found to be an indissoluble and unavoidable relationship with the other. To reconstruct the social bonds means to retrieve the lacking subject, the subject of lack, and the constitutional need for the other.

Colucci, in the above definition, avoids the term 'community', which Basaglia recurrently uses, and I believe this to be a deliberate omission, in that the term has come to signify something rather different from what Basaglia originally had in mind. In psychiatry, the meaning of the 'overused' concept of community (Acheson, 1985: 3) is decided by its dictionary definition: community 'includes two particularly relevant meanings, which refer both to the people in a particular area and to the locality itself' (Tansella and Thornicroft, 2000: 1547–48). As far as psychiatric intervention and mental health care are concerned, the community is

> a defined population, for whom an integrated system of mental health care can be provided. Such a population may be geographically defined or may be identified by some other key criteria. (Tansella and Thornicroft, 2000: 1548)

The notion of 'population' directly connects with Foucault's conceptualisation of biopolitics, as the definition of 'population' 'made possible a logic in which the government of the state came to involve [both] individualization and totalization' (Curtis, 2002: 510). Defining the notion of population enables Foucault to articulate the 'development of anatomo-political techniques aimed at the individual body [with] the development of biopolitical techniques aimed at the collective or social body' (Curtis, 2002: 506). As Curtis (2002: 510) continues, population entails the definition of an essence common to all the members of the population, which can be therefore expounded only in statistical terms. In the context of psychiatry (and medicine broadly speaking), defining a population, which Tansella and Thornicroft seem to regard as a synonym of defining a community, means to reduce all members to their common traits; that is to say, their human nature being understood as set of universal characteristics. It also reduces the psychological depths of the members of the population to shared mental functions and behaviour, thus actually defining their psychology by means of statistical analysis. In the light of these considerations it is all the more important to understand that the notion of individual does not logically precede that of population but is one of its consequences. Thus, the individual, at least in a biopolitical regime, is the atom of the population; the traits and features of single individuals depend upon the statistical description of the population to which they belong.

If such a definition of community is accepted, Basaglia's position would create a vicious circle: psychiatrists establish an intersubjective relationship with patients that is no longer mediated by the positivist distinction between subject and object; by bracketing mental illness, they try to understand the patient rather than explain the patient's symptoms; and so forth. But in doing so, the psychiatrists' ultimate aim would still be to reintegrate the sick person into a community defined as a population. And if, in a state of biopolitics, power is exerted not on individuals directly but on the entire population defined in statistical terms, then the aim of such psychiatry would be to again return individuals to the space where they would be most effectively woven into relations of power. This is among Rotelli's concerns, which he reveals in 'Quale politica per la salute mentale alla fine di un secolo di riforme?'. He asks:

> di che tipo di comunità dobbiamo parlare per il futuro, posto che di comunità dobbiamo comunque parlare, di relazionalità dobbiamo comunque parlare? [...] Dov'è la comunità, lo spazio in cui noi possiamo portare avanti questa pratica terapeutica che non può non essere fonte di emancipazione? Dov'è il luogo concreto, il sito, dov'è lo strumento per emanciparci ed emancipare, se il muro è crollato e se, al di là di esso, spazi capaci di dar forma al legame sociale non esistono? (Rotelli, 1999: 93–94)

Basaglia's (utopian) notion of community might answer Rotelli's questions, insofar as it cannot be reduced to a definable part of the population. Basaglia's 'community' involves a wider concept than the one I have described so far, and, arguably, anticipates that elaborated in the last two decades in the work of the Italian philosopher Roberto Esposito, one of the most important critics of biopolitics, and also the promoter of a possible affirmative declension of biopolitics.

Affirmative Biopolitics between *Communitas* and *Immunitas*

According to Esposito, community is neither 'un soggetto collettivo' nor an 'insieme di soggetti'; it is 'la relazione che non li fa essere più [...] soggetti individuali' (Esposito, 2008b: 92). In other words, it is a 'ni-ente', a 'nothingness' that subtracts the subject from the 'identità con se stesso' and delivers it to an 'alterità irriducibile' (Esposito, 2008b: 81). People tend to protect themselves from belonging to such a community as this entails a partial loss of their identity and, with it, of their subjectivity:

> gli individui [...] divengono davvero tali [...] solo se preventivamente liberati dal debito che li vincola all'altro. Se esentati [...] da quel contatto che minaccia la loro identità esponendoli al possibile conflitto con il loro vicino. (Esposito, 1998: xxiv)

Individuals tend to avoid the risk of losing their identity and entering in a communitarian relationship understood in these terms. A community, thus, does not amount to a

> moltiplicazione della soggettività per un numero indeterminato di individui così come l'individuo costituirebbe un frammento della comunità che aspetta solo di entrare in rapporto con gli altri per realizzarsi interamente. (Esposito, 1998: 74)

Individuals are not 'independent atoms' of the community, ready to realise themselves upon establishing a relationship with the other. On the contrary, the 'soggetto individuo, indiviso, lungi dall'essere una inconsapevole parte della comunità, è proprio ciò che le sbarra la strada' (Esposito, 1998: 74). According to those terms, there can be no community as long as a strong and substantive notion of individuality dominates the way in which human beings understand themselves. In other words, such a community is one which is founded on the utopian notion of lacking subjects rather than on the dystopian notion of individuality.

The word 'community' comes from the Latin *communitas*, which is composed of *cum-* [with], 'ciò che non è proprio' and *munus*, the gift that 'si dà perché si *deve* dare e *non si può non* dare' (Esposito, 1998: xii, xiv). Esposito (1998: xv) puts forward the notion that community is based not on common property but on a debt; community 'non da un più, ma da un "meno"'. In a community, human beings are in fact expropriated 'della loro proprietà iniziale [...] della loro stessa soggettività' (Esposito, 1998: xvi). Interestingly, Stoppa uses the concept of *munus* to define the 'impegno', the 'mission' of the psychiatrists and social workers who are involved in the continuous process of deinstitutionalisation and contribute to creating communities for mental health care. In his words,

> nel caso della nostra pratica, il *munus* (oggi, più prosaicamente, si usa parlare di *mission*), cioè l'impegno, il dono che gli operatori portano a favore dell'umanizzazione delle istituzioni, è rappresentato dal loro pensiero prima e dalla loro azione poi (azione dove la passione deve sposare la cautela, il desiderio, la misura). (Stoppa, 2006: 30)

The resistance towards the formation of a communitarian relationship is connected to the notion of 'immunity'. According to Esposito, in the contemporary capitalist society we are witnessing what he calls an excess of immunity, which hinders the formation of a community, and promotes a negative – thanatopolitical – drift in biopolitics. *Immunitas* (literally, immunity) might seem to be the exact opposite of community: it is the avoidance of the *munus*, of the debt, the lack that preempts the possibility of a communitarian relationship. On the one hand, *immunitas* is the 'autonomia originaria o [...] sollevamento successivo da un debito precedentemente contratto' (Esposito, 2002: 8): those who are immune are exempted from the *munus* that would introduce them to the community. It is therefore something radically anti-social, 'e più precisamente anti-comunitario'. In exempting the subject from the obligation of a reciprocal donation, it also 'interrompe il circuito sociale' (Esposito, 2002: 9). Nonetheless, Esposito (2002: 9) adds a second interpretation of immunity, which draws on biomedical language: according to this, immunity is the 'condizione di refrattarietà dell'organismo rispetto al pericolo di contrarre una malattia'. This concept entered the biomedical vocabulary during the eighteenth and nineteenth centuries, especially with the discovery of vaccinations and bacteriology. Hence, *immunitas* is tied to a process of reaction to the external world, bacteria and other possible vectors of contagion. But any process of immunisation, for instance, vaccinations, implies 'la presenza del male che deve contrastare': 'il male va contrastato – ma non tenendolo lontano dai propri confini. Al contrario, includendolo all'interno di essi' (Esposito, 2002: 10). Hence, there is no community without a certain amount of immunity. In the same way as the human body, the community needs some level of protection and immunisation: on a macro-social level, this is a condition of affirmative biopolitics. The social body is barely immunised from the outside and from the inside, it is 'porous'.

The problems begin when there is an *excess* of immunisation. In medicine, this happens, for instance, where there is a reversal in the target of antibodies: the organism develops an auto-immune syndrome such as lupus. The body fights against itself, in that 'l'immunità, necessaria a proteggere la nostra vita, se portata oltre una certa soglia, finisce per negarla' (Esposito, 2005: 161). On a macro-social level, this is the opposite of an affirmative biopolitics; it is thanatopolitics, an exertion of ruthless biopower. The most often used (and indeed most extreme) example of this is, of course, as noted in Chapter 5, Nazi Germany: the politics of immunisation (eugenics to defend the pure race, for instance) turn against the social body itself.

In short, immunisation grounds the process of individualisation: individuals immunise themselves from their constitutional lack and from the 'possibilità dissolutiva della "messa in comune"' (Esposito, 2002: 18). Whilst this is, to a certain extent, a necessary part in the formation of a community – the creation of a gap, a distance, between the subject and the other – an excess of immunisation halts the community, which comes to be felt as a threat to subjectivity, as the ultimate limit to its (illusory) wholeness.

From these considerations, it should become clear that Basaglia's entire *oeuvre* can be read in the light of Esposito's notion of 'immunisation'. The state of *alienità* corresponds to an excess of immunisation that hinders the possibility of establishing a communitarian relationship. Yet a certain, limited amount of immunisation must be in place to grant subjectivity a minimum of separation from otherness – as shown in Chapter 2, Basaglia calls it the *intervallo*. Without such a gap the lived body, the threshold between subjectivity and otherness, could not emerge. When this negotiated *intervallo* does not become a hiatus, and thus does not get in the way of the intersubjective relationship, then there is a state of proper *alterità* which, in Esposito's terms, would correspond to a communitarian relationship, to the *communitas* – a 'space' where the subject comes into being as lacking.

What is more, Foucault's own concept of 'graft' can be read as a paradigm of immunisation. If there is a graft, a *nodo*, between madness and reason, this is because madness must be rationalised in order for it not to represent a threat to rationality. Only when madness is completely reduced to mental illness, to a rational construct, can there be a science entrusted with its elimination, that is, with protecting society and individuals from the possible negative consequences of madness: rationality immunises itself against madness, the social body immunises itself against social deviants, etc.

The paradigm of immunisation is implicit in Foucault's conceptualisation of graft as early as *History of Madness*, in which he affirms that madness meets the medical gaze because people fear that it may be contagious (Foucault, 2006a: 355). And it is implicit in all of his work on psychiatry, especially when, in *Abnormal*, he acknowledges the shift from assistance of the sick person to protection of society (Foucault, 2006b: 220), sanctioning the 'enthronement' of psychiatry as an apparatus of immunisation.

It is with reference to the introduction of the therapeutic community into psychiatry practice that Basaglia thoroughly conceptualises the notion of 'community' (as opposed to the notion of 'subject', which he never clearly defines). His main inspiration is the work of the American phenomenological psychologist Erling Eng, and especially his paper 'Body, We-awareness, and Therapeutic Community' (1968), which Basaglia recursively cites in his paper 'Corpo e istituzione'. According to Eng (1968: 184, quoted in Basaglia, 1967a: 113), community is 'simply the immediate sense of shared experience as this is present in facing one another. It is a directly grasped understanding. [...] It is, in the fullest sense "we-awareness"'. Such 'we-awareness' is, according to Basaglia (1967a: 112), pre-reflexive, in that 'nasce direttamente dal fatto di essere-insieme'. Once again, it is clear from such statements that, according to Basaglia, intersubjectivity logically and ontogenetically precedes subjectivity. What is more, this pre-reflexive 'essere-insieme' also shapes, according to Eng – and to Basaglia – the 'lived body': thrown into the world as the 'object' of the other, the body becomes the pole through which I am able to perceive myself as a subject, to become a subject. Thanks to the exposed and fragile presence of the body in the world, I am able to actively become a subject through the shaping action of the other: the body is the threshold between subjectivity and otherness.

Insofar as one accepts and establishes such an indissoluble, constitutive and constitutional link between subjectivity, otherness and the body, a communitarian relationship can be said to have come into being, and, with it, the subject as lacking. According to both Eng and Basaglia, what used to happen in psychiatry was that the 'lived body' (Eng calls it the 'own body') tended to be disregarded in favour of flattening the patient's experience of the body onto the 'anatomical', sick, body. Eng (1968: 185–86) says:

> If we start with 'community' as we-awareness, we can recover the 'own body' which so often becomes lost from sight for both patient and doctor during the development and treatment of psychiatrically-defined illness. Nor is it sufficient to point out that the psychiatric patient has lost touch with his 'own body' to justify his treatment as bodily in the object sense. In any event, the evidence [...] seems compelling that it is from a matrix of lived community that the own body emerges.

Understood in such a way, therefore, the community is that intersubjective *a priori* in which the lived body emerges and, with it, a subjectivity that is intrinsically connected and constitutionally second to intersubjectivity. This should not, however, lead us to infer that 'what we call "society" is simply generative of the individual', because the communitarian relationship, understood in these terms, 'precedes the constitution of society as such. The community that is prior to the realisation of the own body is insufficiently differentiated to be considered as a causal agent' (Eng, 1968: 186).

According to Basaglia (1967a: 113), these considerations should ground the very implementation of the therapeutic community, which should be

> una comunità che si fondi sulla interazione preriflessiva di tutti i suoi membri; dove il rapporto non sia il rapporto oggettivante del signore con il servo, o di chi dà e chi riceve; dove tutti i membri della comunità possano – attraverso la contestazione reciproca e la dialettizzazione delle reciproche posizioni – ricostruire il proprio corpo proprio e il proprio ruolo.

This – 'properly' – therapeutic community could be regarded as the basis for establishing a different dialectical relationship between the patient and the psychiatrist, between the subject and the institution, and, perhaps, even between the individual and society, which it would do by highlighting the indissoluble relationship that exists between the intersubjective dimension, subjectivity, the lived and the organic body:

> La dialettica fra individuo e organizzazione dovrebbe esprimersi come dialettica fra un corpo organico che risulti appropriato dal soggetto nella sua organicità al gruppo, quindi organico alla costruzione delle risposte ai bisogni propri e del gruppo; e un corpo sociale che risulti la somma di soggetti partecipi alla propria organizzazione e all'organizzazione delle risposte ai bisogni propri e del gruppo. Corpo organico e corpo sociale sarebbero, in questo caso, espressione di una soggettività individuale contenuta in una soggettività collettiva. Ma il sistema produttivo che è venuto affermandosi si fonda sull'appropriazione della soggettività dell'uomo, quindi sulla riduzione del corpo organico a corpo e sulla tendenziale identificazione fra corpo sociale e corpo economico. (Basaglia, 1979a: 427)

In the context of psychiatry, and especially in the context of institutional psychiatry, a community understood in these terms can only be *rebuilt*, neglected and disregarded as it was in the asylum of old and in the humanised psychiatric hospital. However, Basaglia's notion of community does not exhaust its revolutionary potentiality even *after* the era of the psychiatric hospital; that is to say, in a state of advanced biopolitics where, in the context of psychiatry at least, the notion of community and that of population seem to overlap.

Basaglia's Holistic Approach: An Affirmative Biopolitical Psychiatry?

The term, *polis*, that Colucci uses suggests a broader level than the one which is usually tackled in clinical psychiatry. According the classification of social interventions by Lehtinen et al. (2007: 137) working, even theoretically, at the level of the *polis* would entail a macro-social intervention. Indeed, according to Basaglia this is (or at least was, during the struggle against the asylum and institutional psychiatry) one of the most important levels of action, the site where alternative psychiatrists could really make a difference. However, the macro-social level cannot be faced without interventions also at a meso-social (the organisation of the actual places catering for mental health care), and micro-social level (the patient's families and affections). And, in turn, micro-social interventions would not be possible without a 'clinic of the subject', otherwise, there would once again be a complete disregard for the patients themselves.

What should be central to any psychiatric intervention, according to Basaglia, more than anything else, is a holistic approach, capable of simultaneously tackling the several different aspects that mental disorders entail. Let us take the example of institutional and disciplinary psychiatry. The subjectivity of inmates in the asylum is disregarded: their alleged diagnosed illnesses would be the exclusive focus of attention, and intervention inside the asylum would aim at making patients as manageable as possible. The conditions of inmates, however, do not derive from their subjective experience, although, possibly, they might have been referred to the asylum by their families or closest friends (micro-social level). In response to the family's call, society would have provided a specific place, organised in a certain way, to cope with the issue (the asylum, meso-social level), and this kind of reaction would depend on social norms and widespread 'scientific' beliefs (that a certain behaviour is scandalous, that mentally ill people can be dangerous to themselves or to others, that isolation in the asylum could be a treatment in itself, etc.) (macro-social level). A psychiatrist who wants to change this pattern should act on all levels: in the intersubjective relationship with the patient – because mental disorders do exist and the patient is indeed suffering; in the relationship at a micro-social level – for instance, to explain to the family that the patient is not dangerous after all; in the organisation of the services provided – for instance, allowing asylum inmates to go off the premises, or abolishing the asylum *tout court*; and finally, at a macro-social level, intervening to change social norms, and the widespread beliefs concerning mental illness. Acting on one or few levels only, as Basaglia has shown, would not prove particularly effective: one can abolish the straitjacket, but with the asylum still standing the inmate would still be locked away; one can reintegrate the former inmate into society, but society would still be structured around a productive cycle which has no space for the former inmate, and so on.

Basaglia's holistic approach derives from a complex theoretical framework and entails clinical interventions at subjective, organic, intersubjective, micro-, meso-, and macro-social levels. The elements of such a complex theoretical framework, which extends from the phenomenological/existentialist theory of the subject to a Foucauldian criticism of social normativity, yet without neglecting the organicity and biological nature of the human body, and the numerous levels of proposed clinical intervention, can be reduced to the interplay between the above discussed notions of subject as lacking and of community as *communitas*. A psychiatric praxis – utopian as it might be – read in the light of these notions should be understood in terms of a communitarian relationship.

The community Basaglia argues for is based on the concept of *alterità*, which entails acknowledging not only the distance between the subject and the other but also and especially the unavoidability of the relationship with the other. Subjects thus do not fall into a state of *alienità*, which, as we have seen, means to lose the distance from the other and fade into it. To rebuild a community means to recover a constitutional lack, to recognise that the subject 'è caratterizzato da una mancanza originaria che non può riempire' (Esposito, 2007: 135): this constitutional lack is consubstantial with the need for the other. Therapy does not aim at recuperating an (illusory) substantial subjectivity or, better still, individuality, as would be the case, say, in approaches such as ego psychology or even the more recent empowerment psychotherapy. The ultimate result of these approaches would be to strengthen the alienation of the patient into a notion of individuality, which is itself the effect of power relations and forms of societal control.

A 'clinic of the subject' moves from the idea that the subject is constitutionally lacking, an idea that Basaglia formulated as early as his 1953 article, 'Il mondo dell'incomprensibile schizofrenico'. In this article, he claimed for the first time that the subject cannot establish a direct relationship with itself; that is, a reflexive relationship, if one is not in a relationship with the other. We have also seen that Basaglia's primary concern in his early work was to define a method, which he found in *Daseinsanalyse*, capable of accounting for both the psychiatrist's and the patient's subjectivities, as opposed to the positivist subject-object relationship. Basaglia's early conception of the relationship between the patient and the psychiatrist already entails a communitarian relationship: both psychiatrist and patient call into question their own subjectivities and structure the relationship around their constitutional lack – to a certain extent, they embrace the primacy of intersubjectivity over subjectivity. To this extent, to reject a paradigm of immunisation in psychiatry would mean to 'accettare il conflitto che ogni soggetto produce, senza difendersi dietro schemi interpretativi diventati ormai dogmi' (Ongaro Basaglia, 1998): in other words, 'bracketing' mental illness, establishing an intersubjective relationship, entering this relationship 'disarmati' (Basaglia, 1979b: 307), refusing the traditional role of psychiatrist. In short, the condition of ideological void left by the implementation of Law 180 could be read in this light: as an attempt at contrasting the paradigms of immunisation and establishing, if not a community understood in the above terms, at least the possibility for such a communitarian relationship to come into being.

This utopian community is not an ideal world 'dove tutti sono buoni, dove i rapporti sono improntati al più profondo umanitarismo, dove il lavoro risulti gratificante' (Basaglia, 1997: 20) but should be understood in terms of what Esposito calls a 'democrazia porosa'; that is to say, a democracy in which power relations and paradigms of immunisation are not completely erased (because it would not be possible), but 'le cui forme siano sempre oggetto di innovazione e autosuperamento' (Esposito, 2008a: 26). Basaglia himself observes that, in defining a communitarian relationship, it is not possible to completely avoid power relations and paradigms of immunisation: the critical characteristic of a 'properly' therapeutic community is its ability to be guided and not determined by relations of power, a community capable of overcoming itself and constantly referring to the needs of it members. In Basaglia's words,

> problema sarà quello del come organizzare una comunità che non deve essere determinata, che non può essere comandata ma solo diretta da un potere che sappia limitarsi ad instradarla e a coordinarne le forze. (Basaglia, 1966b: 63)

That is to say, the community is to be understood as 'un abbozzo di sistema cui riferirsi, per subito trascenderlo e distruggerlo' (Basaglia, 1966b: 63). As Stoppa (2006: 29) contends, community is a 'realtà mai compiuta, "possibile" [...], che richiede un costante lavoro di manutenzione'.

The notions of *communitas*, *immunitas* and also that of 'democrazia porosa' contribute to forming, according to Esposito, the outline of a potential affirmative biopolitical scenario, understood as a possible 'way out' of Foucault's oscillations, which engendered 'due tonalità [...] opposte' in interpreting biopolitics: 'una radicalmente negativa [...] e l'altra marcatamente affermativa, quasi euforica' (Esposito, 2005: 158). If, in fact, it is not the case that life can be 'salvata dalla politica', it is, on the contrary, the case that politics might be 'ripensata a partire da quella vita da cui è sempre stata implicata anche quando ha preteso di farla propria e di dirigerla ai propri fini' (Esposito, 2005: 163). Esposito sees in 'birth' the ontology of such rethinking, of this affirmative biopolitical scenario, where life – 'intesa nella sua irriducibile complessità, come un fenomeno pluridimensionale che in un certo senso va sempre aldilà di se stesso' (Esposito, 2005: 163–64) – shapes politics without being negatively controlled and thanatopolitically 'disallowed to the point of death' (Foucault, 1998: 138). Pregnancy gives an example of how two immune systems can coexist and strengthen each other to foster life: the relationship between mother and baby is, according to Esposito, the perfect example of a *communitas*. *Immunitas* is not absent, because there would be no life without a certain level of immunisation; however, 'la nascita costituisce il punto originario in cui l'*immunitas* fa tutt'uno con la *communitas* – in cui la prima non neutralizza, ma potenzia e amplifica la seconda' (Esposito, 2005: 166). Certainly, the ultimate outcomes of Esposito's affirmative biopolitics are questionable and they have indeed been subjected to strong criticism: Chiesa (2011) contends that Esposito, by placing birth as the point of origin of an affirmative biopolitics and by sanctioning its 'obligatoriness', eventually comes to theorise a metaphysics of life not dissimilar to religious pro-life stances. Thus, in grounding an affirmative biopolitics on the 'ontological obligatoriness' of birth, Esposito seems to be *de facto* reproducing the same metaphysical premises that engender thanatopolitical drifts.

Nevertheless, we do not need to follow Esposito to the extreme fringes of his thought in order to recognise in Basaglia's utopian notions of community and subjectivity the embryonic conception of, if not a possible affirmative biopolitical psychiatry then a psychiatry that does not endorse, and even actively opposes, the immunitarian and thanatopolitical drifts of contemporary biopolitics. Di Vittorio, and, with him, most critics of contemporary (Italian) psychiatry, tend to assume, or, at least this is what transpires from their works, that a state of biopolitics is negative *per se*, especially in the context of mental health care, where it seems to reproduce the abuses that had emerged in the era of disciplinary and institutional psychiatry – coercive and punitive measures, unjustified limits to the freedom of patients/inmates, creation of docile and subjugated patients/inmates/individuals, and so forth. At the same time, they highlight new risks and negative effects specific to a 'biopolitical' psychiatry: the creation of fragile individuals, constantly perceiving themselves as being 'at risk' (of mental disorders, for instance), incapable of dealing with normal albeit painful states such as bereavement, always in need of support by a plethora of pedagogues, psychiatrists, psychologists, learning technologists, counsellors, etc.; the creation of new but equally alienating 'patterns of normality' and normativity based on statistical studies; the extensive use of psychopharmacology in all sorts of non-medical ways; the flattening of the psychosocial onto the biological; the list could go on. All this is clearly regarded as a 'betrayal' of Basaglia's legacy. His work of reform, allegedly aimed at eliminating the institutionalising and coercive aspect of psychiatry – a medical science which has been often used as an instrument of social control – is regarded as not entirely successful because it failed to oppose the rise of such a negative 'biopolitical' psychiatry. This position is not entirely wrong and, as I have shown in the previous chapter, all the negative elements of the state of biopolitics that have been enumerated are real concerns, and indeed should not be ignored, especially by policymakers in the context of mental health care. However, demonising biopolitics and, in the specific examples tackled in this book, its effect on psychiatry, casts too dark a shadow on the actual positive outcomes, not only of Italian psychiatric reform but also and especially of psychiatry as a medical science.

If there is a 'contenuto reale' of the alternative psychiatry proposed by Basaglia, then I believe it could be regarded as a holistic approach to mental health care, capable, possibly through the employment of multidisciplinary teams, of dealing with the numerous and different aspects that mental disorders entail. Such an approach is not distant, at least on paper and almost exclusively in high-income countries, from how psychiatry is indeed practised at a clinical level, and how it is envisioned by policymakers. This does not mean that there is no room for improvement, especially at the level of implementation, and the state of affairs is certainly far from idyllic. However, demonising it *tout court* makes of 'sventolare il libretto rosso' an empty gesture, while it could, and should, rather be brought to represent a heightened critical attention towards the looming thanatopolitical drift of any biopolitics. In psychiatry as much as in medicine in general and in many other branches of knowledge, the tension between biopolitics and thanatopolitics, the two faces of the co-implication between politics and life, cannot be ignored. Basaglia seems to anticipate a way to understand this co-implication and its consequences in the context of psychiatry: the ontology of subjectivity and community that he proposes paves the way to a possible affirmative declension of biopolitical psychiatry, beyond its all too easy demonisation and its enthusiastic adoption.

Bibliography

Abboud, L. (2005). 'The Next Phase in Psychiatry'. *The Wall Street Journal*, 27 July. Available at <http://online.wsj.com/article/0,,SB112242117930696793,00.html>, accessed 15 March 2012.

Abraham, K. (1927). 'A Short Study of the Development of the Libido, Viewed in the Light of Mental Disorders'. Translated by Douglas Bryan and Alix Strachey. In: *Selected Papers on Psycho-Analysis*. London: Hogarth, pp. 418–79.

Acheson, E.D. (1985). 'That Over-Used Word Community'. *Health Trends*, 17, p. 3.

Agamben, G. (2003). *Stato di eccezione*. Turin: Bollati Boringhieri.

—— (2005). *Homo sacer: Il potere sovrano e la nuda vita*. Turin: Einaudi.

Allaby, M. (2006). 'Graft'. Available at <http://www.oxfordreference.com/views/ENTRY.html?subview=Main&entry=t7.e3018>, accessed 17 March 2009.

Almeida-Filho, N., et al. (1997). 'Brazilian Multicentric Study of Psychiatric Morbidity'. *British Journal of Psychiatry*, 171, pp. 524–29.

Andreasen, N. (1997). 'Linking Mind and Brain in the Study of Mental Illness: A Project for a Scientific Psychopathology'. *Science*, 5306, pp. 1586–93.

Andrews, G., et al. (2001). 'Prevalence, Comorbidity, Disability and Service Utilisation: Overview of the Australian National Mental Health Survey'. *British Journal of Psychiatry*, 178, pp. 145–53.

APA (1968). *Diagnostic and Statistical Manual of Mental Disorders* (2nd edn). Washington, DC: American Psychiatric Press.

—— (2000). *Diagnostic and Statistical Manual of Mental Disorders, Text Revision* (4th edn). Washington, DC: American Psychiatric Press.

Armocida, G. (2007). 'A.M. Fiamberti and "Psycosurgery"'. *Medicina nei secoli*, 19(2), pp. 457–74.

Armstrong, D. (1995). 'Bodies of Knowledge/Knowledge of Bodies'. In: Jones, C., and Porter, R. (eds), *Reassessing Foucault: Power, Medicine and the Body*. London: Routledge, pp. 17–27.

—— (1997). 'Foucault and the Sociology of Health and Illness'. In: Petersen, A., and Burton, R. (eds), *Foucault, Health and Medicine*. London: Routledge, pp. 15–30.

Artaud, A. (1947). 'Van Gogh. The Man Suicided by Society'. In: Hirshman, J. (ed.), *Antonin Artaud Anthology*. San Francisco: City Light Books (1965), pp. 135–63.

Balduzzi, E., et al. (1979). *Il giardino dei gelsi*. Turin: Einaudi.

Barbui, C., et al. (1999). 'QUALYOP Project 2: Monitoring the Dismantling of Italian Psychiatric Hospitals. Psychotropic Drug Use in 1,072 Inpatients'. *Pharmacoepidemiology and Drug Safety*, 8, pp. 331–37.

Barham, P. (1992). 'Foucault and the Psychiatric Practitioner'. In: Still, A., and Velody, I. (eds), *Rewriting the History of Madness*. London: Routledge, pp. 45–50.

Barton, R. (1959). *Institutional Neurosis*. Bristol: John Wright.

Basaglia, F. (1952). 'Esposizione di alcuni casi di utile impiego del test del disegno nei disturbi del linguaggio, Comunicazione alla sezione Veneto-Emiliana di Neurologia'. *Rivista Sperimentale di Freniatria*, 76(f2).

—— (1953a). 'Il mondo dell'"incomprensibile" schizofrenico attraverso la "Daseinsanalyse". Presentazione di un caso clinico'. In: Basaglia, F., *Scritti*, ed. Ongaro Basaglia, Vol. 1. Turin: Einaudi, 1981, pp. 3–54.

—— (1953b). 'Sull'impiego del test di associazione verbale secondo Rapaport in clinica psichiatrica, Riassunto della comunicazione svolta alla sezione Veneto-Emiliana di Neurologia'. *Rivista di neurologia*, 23(f6).

—— (1954a). 'Contributo allo studio psicopatologico e clinico degli stati ossessivi'. In: Basaglia, F., *Scritti*, ed. Ongaro Basaglia, Vol. 1. Turin: Einaudi, 1981, pp. 55–103.

—— (1954b). 'Su alcuni aspetti della moderna psicoterapia: Analisi fenomenologica dell'"incontro"'. In: Basaglia, F., *Scritti*, ed. Ongaro Basaglia, Vol. 1. Turin: Einaudi, 1981, pp. 32–54.

—— (1956a). 'Il corpo nell'ipocondria e nella depersonalizzazione. La coscienza del corpo e il sentimento di esistenza corporea nella depersonalizzazione somatopsichica'. In: Basaglia, F., *Scritti*, ed. Ongaro Basaglia, Vol. 1. Turin: Einaudi, 1981, pp. 165–206.

—— (1956b). 'Il corpo nell'ipocondria e nella depersonalizzazione. La struttura psicopatologica dell'ipocondria'. In: Basaglia, F., *Scritti*, ed. Ongaro Basaglia, *Scritti*, Vol. 1, Turin: Einaudi, 1981, pp. 137–64.

—— (1957). 'L'ipocondria come deformazione dell'"Erlebnis" individuale nel fenomeno di depersonalizzazione'. In: Basaglia, F., *Scritti*, ed. Ongaro Basaglia, Vol. 1. Turin: Einaudi, 1981, pp. 104–11.

—— (1963). 'Ansia e malafede. La condizione umana del nevrotico'. In: Basaglia, F., *L'utopia della realtà*, ed. Ongaro Basaglia. Turin: Einaudi, 2005, pp. 3–16.

—— (1964a). 'La distruzione dell'ospedale psichiatrico come luogo di istituzionalizzazione'. In: Basaglia, F., *L'utopia della realtà*, ed. Ongaro Basaglia. Turin: Einaudi, 2005, pp. 17–26.

—— (1964b). 'La libertà comunitaria come alternativa alla regressione istituzionale'. In: Basaglia, F., *Scritti*, ed. Ongaro Basaglia, Vol. 1. Turin: Einaudi, 1981, pp. 394–409.

—— (1965a). 'Corpo, sguardo e silenzio. L'enigma della soggettività in psichiatria'. In: Basaglia, F., *L'utopia della realtà*, ed. Ongaro Basaglia. Turin: Einaudi, 2005, pp. 27–42.

—— (1965b). 'La "comunità terapeutica" come base di un servizio psichiatrico'. In: Basaglia, F., *Scritti*, ed. Ongaro Basaglia, Vol. 1. Turin: Einaudi, 1981, pp. 259–82.

—— (1965c). 'Potere ed istituzionalizzazione. Dalla vita istituzionale alla vita di comunità'. In: Basaglia, F., *Scritti*, ed. Ongaro Basaglia, Vol. 1. Turin: Einaudi, 1981, pp. 283–93.

—— (1966a). 'L'ideologia del corpo come espressività nevrotica'. In: Basaglia, F., *L'utopia della realtà*, ed. Ongaro Basaglia. Turin: Einaudi, 2005, pp. 64–99.

—— (1966b). 'Un problema di psichiatria istituzionale'. In: Basaglia, F., *L'utopia della realtà*, ed. Ongaro Basaglia. Turin: Einaudi, 2005, pp. 43–63.

—— (1967a). 'Corpo e istituzione. Considerazioni antropologiche e psicopatologiche in tema di psichiatria istituzionale'. In: Basaglia, F., *L'utopia della realtà*, ed. Ongaro Basaglia. Turin: Einaudi, 2005, pp. 100–13.

—— (1967b). 'Crisi istituzionale o crisi psichiatrica?'. In: Basaglia, F., *L'utopia della realtà*, ed. Ongaro Basaglia, Turin: Einaudi, 2005, pp. 114–26.

—— (1967c). 'Esclusione, programmazione e integrazione. Appunti sulla realtà psichiatrica italiana'. In: Basaglia, F., *Scritti*, ed. Ongaro Basaglia, Vol. 1. Turin: Einaudi, 1981, pp. 410–23.

—— (1967d). 'La soluzione finale'. In: Basaglia, F., *L'utopia della realtà*, ed. Ongaro Basaglia. Turin: Einaudi, 2005, pp. 138–47.

—— (1968a). 'Il problema della gestione'. In: Basaglia, F., *Scritti*, ed. Ongaro Basaglia, Vol. 1, Turin: Einaudi, 1981, pp. 512–21.

—— (1968b). 'La comunità terapeutica e le istituzioni psichiatriche'. In: Basaglia, F., *Scritti*, ed. Ongaro Basaglia, Vol. 2. Turin: Einaudi, 1981, pp. 3–13.

—— (1968c). 'Le istituzioni della violenza'. In: Basaglia, F., *Scritti*, ed. Ongaro Basaglia, Vol. 1. Turin: Einaudi, 1981, pp. 471–505.

—— (1968d). 'Le istituzioni della violenza e le istituzioni della tolleranza'. In: Basaglia, F., *Scritti*, ed. Ongaro Basaglia, Vol. 2, Turin: Einaudi, 1981, pp. 80–95.

—— (1968e). 'Prefazione a "L'istituzione negata"'. In: Basaglia, F., *Scritti*, ed. Ongaro Basaglia, Vol. 1. Turin: Einaudi, 1981, pp. 468–70.

—— (1968f). 'Relazione alla commissione di studio per l'aggiornamento delle vigenti norme sulle costruzioni ospedaliere'. In: Basaglia, F., *Scritti*, ed. Ongaro Basaglia, Vol. 2. Turin: Einaudi, 1981, pp. 14–32.

—— (1969a). 'Introduzione ad "Asylums"'. In: Basaglia, F., *Scritti*, ed. Ongaro Basaglia, Vol. 2. Turin: Einaudi, 1981, pp. 33–46.

—— (1969b). 'Lettera da New York. Il malato artificiale'. In: Basaglia, F., *L'utopia della realtà*, ed. Ongaro Basaglia. Turin: Einaudi, 2005, pp. 182–91.

—— (1970a). 'La malattia e il suo doppio. Proposte critiche sul problema delle devianze'. In: Basaglia, F., *Scritti*, ed. Ongaro Basaglia, Vol. 2. Turin: Einaudi, 1981, pp. 126–46.

—— (1970b). 'Prefazione a "Ideologia e pratica della psichiatria sociale"'. In: Basaglia, F., *Scritti*, ed. Ongaro Basaglia, Vol. 2. Turin: Einaudi, 1981, pp. 105–25.

—— (1971a). 'La giustizia che punisce. Appunti sull'ideologia della punizione'. In: Basaglia, F., *Scritti*, ed. Ongaro Basaglia, Vol. 2. Turin: Einaudi, 1981, pp. 185–98.

—— (1971b). 'Riabilitazione e controllo sociale'. In: Basaglia, F., *Scritti*, ed. Ongaro Basaglia, Vol. 2. Turin: Einaudi, 1981, pp. 199–208.

—— (1973). 'Prefazione a "La marchesa e i demoni"'. In: Basaglia, F., *Scritti*, ed. Ongaro Basaglia, Vol. 2. Turin: Einaudi, 1981, pp. 209–21.

—— (1975a). 'Crimini di pace'. In: Basaglia, F., *Scritti*, ed. Ongaro Basaglia, Vol. 2. Turin: Einaudi, 1981, pp. 237–338.

—— (1975b). 'Ideologia e pratica in tema di salute mentale'. In: Basaglia, F., *Scritti*, ed. Ongaro Basaglia, Vol. 2. Turin: Einaudi, 1981, pp. 354–61.

—— (1976). 'La giustizia che non riesce a difendere se stessa'. In: Basaglia, F., *Scritti*, ed. Ongaro Basaglia, Vol. 2. Turin: Einaudi, 1981, pp. 382–90.

—— (1977). 'Il circuito del controllo: Dal manicomio al decentramento psichiatrico'. In: Basaglia, F., *Scritti*, ed. Ongaro Basaglia, Vol. 2. Turin: Einaudi, 1981, pp. 391–410.

—— (1978a). 'Che dice Basaglia'. *La Stampa*, 12 May 1978, p. 11.

—— (1978b). 'Introduzione a "Lo Psicanalismo"'. In: Basaglia, F., *Scritti*, ed. Ongaro Basaglia, Vol. 2. Turin: Einaudi, 1981, pp. 349–53.

—— (1979a). 'Follia/delirio'. In: Basaglia, F., *Scritti*, ed. Ongaro Basaglia, Vol. 2. Turin: Einaudi, 1981, pp. 411–44.

—— (1979b). 'Prefazione a "Il giardino dei Gelsi"'. In: Basaglia, F., *L'utopia della realtà*, ed. Ongaro Basaglia, Turin: Einaudi, 2005, pp. 302–8.

—— (1979c). 'Presentazione inedita'. In: Dell'Acqua, G. (2007), *Non ho l'arma che uccide il leone*. Viterbo: Stampa Alternativa, pp. 4–6.

—— (1980). 'Conversazione: A proposito della nuova legge 180'. In: Basaglia, F., *Scritti*, ed. Ongaro Basaglia, Vol. 2, Turin: Einaudi, 1981, pp. 473–85.

—— (1981a). 'Introduzione generale ed esposizione riassuntiva dei vari gruppi di lavori'. In: Basaglia, F., *Scritti*, ed. Ongaro Basaglia, Vol. 1. Turin: Einaudi, 1981, pp. xix–xliv.

—— (ed.) (1997). *Che cos'è la psichiatria?* Milan: Baldini Castoldi Dalai.

—— (2000). *Conferenze brasiliane*. Milan: Cortina Raffaello.

Basaglia, F., and Ongaro Basaglia, F. (eds) (1971). *La maggioranza deviante*. Turin: Einaudi.

Basaglia, F., and Rigotti, S. (1952). 'Sull'impiego di alcune tecniche proiettive in subnarcosi barbiturica'. *Il Cervello*, 28(5).

Basaglia, F., et al. (1978). *La nave che affonda*, Rome: Savelli.
Basso, E. (2007). *Michel Foucault e la Daseinsanalyse. Un'indagine fenomenologica.* Udine: Mimesis.
Bateman, A.W., and Fonagy, P. (2000). 'Effectiveness of Psychotherapeutic Treatment of Personality Disorder'. *British Journal of Psychiatry*, 177, pp. 138–43.
Battie, W. (1758). *A Treatise on Madness.* London: Whiston.
Bazzicalupo, L. (2010). *Biopolitica. Una mappa concettuale.* Rome: Carocci.
Beaulieu, A. (2006). 'The Hybrid Character of "Control" in the Work of Michel Foucault'. In: Beaulieu, A. and Gabbard, D. (eds), *Michel Foucault and Power Today: International Multidisciplinary Studies in the History of the Present.* Oxford: Lexington Books, pp. 23–34.
Beers, C. (1908). *A Mind That Found Itself.* Pittsburgh: University of Pittsburgh Press.
Begley, S. (2007). 'How Thinking Can Change the Brain'. *The Wall Street Journal*, 19 January 2007, p. B1.
Bentham, J. (1838). *The Works of Jeremy Bentham, published under the superintendence of his executor, John Bowring.* Edinburgh: William Tait.
Benvenuto, S. (2005). 'Psichiatria e critica della tecnica. Franco Basaglia e il movimento psichiatrico anti-istituzionale in Italia'. *Psichiatria e psicoterapia*, XIXV(3), pp. 186–96.
Berlincioni, V., and Petrella, F. (2008). 'Michel Foucault e lo psichiatra'. In: Galzigna, M. (ed.), *Foucault, Oggi.* Milan: Feltrinelli, pp. 106–33.
Bernstein, E., and Dooren, J.C. (2007). 'Antidepressants Get a Boost for Use in Teens'. *The Wall Street Journal*, 18 April 2007, pp. D1, D4.
Bertani, M. (2004). 'La nascita della psichiatria dallo spirito della follia. Nota storica su "Il potere psichiatrico"'. *aut aut*, 323, pp. 52–86.
Bijl, R.V., et al. (1998). 'Prevalence of Psychiatric Disorder in the General Population: Results of the Netherlands Mental Health Survey and Incidence Study (NEMESIS)'. *Social Psychiatry and Psychiatric Epidemiology*, 33(12), pp. 587–95.
Binswanger, L. (1957a). *Der Mensch in der Psychiatrie*, Pfullingen: Neske.
—— (1957b). *Sigmund Freud: Reminiscences of a Friendship.* Translated by Norbert Guterman. New York: Grune and Stratton.
—— (1962). 'Freud's Conception of Man in the Light of Anthropology'. In: Needleman, J. (ed.), *Being-in-the-World. Selected Papers of Ludwig Binswanger.* Translated by Jacob Needleman. London: Basic Books, pp. 149–81.
Bland, R.C., et al. (eds) (1994). 'Epidemiology of Psychiatric Disorders in Edmonton: Phenomenology and Comorbidity'. *Acta Psychiatrica Scandinavica*, Supplement, 376, pp. 1–70.
Blumhagen, D.W. (1979). 'The Doctor's White Coat: The Image of the Physician in Modern America'. *Annals of Internal Medicine*, 91, pp. 111–16.

Bo, R. (2012). 'Gli ex primari: pazienti legati ai letti'. *Gazzetta di Mantova*, 1 August 2012, p. 11.
Bonnie, R. (2002). 'Political Abuse of Psychiatry in the Soviet Union and in China: Complexities and Controversies'. *Journal of the American Academy of Psychiatry and the Law*, 30(1), pp. 136–44.
Bourgois, P. (2000). 'Disciplining Addictions: The Bio-Politics of Methadone and Heroin in the United States'. *Culture, Medicine and Psychiatry*, 24, pp. 165–95.
Boyne, R. (1990). *Foucault and Derrida: The Other Side of Reason*, London: Unwin Hyman.
Braun, B. (2007). 'Biopolitics and the Molecularization of Life'. *Cultural Geographies*, 14, pp. 6–28.
Bühler, K.-E. (2004). 'Existential Analysis and Psychoanalysis: Specific Differences and Personal Relationship Between Ludwig Binswanger and Sigmund Freud'. *American Journal of Psychotherapy*, 58(1), pp. 34–50.
Campbell, R.J. (2009). *Campbell's Psychiatric Dictionary: The Definitive Dictionary of Psychiatry*. Oxford: Oxford University Press.
Canguilhem, G. (2007). *The Normal and the Pathological*. Translated by Carolyn R. Fawcett. New York: Zone Books.
Canosa, R. (1980). *Storia del manicomio in Italia dall'Unità a oggi*. Milan: Feltrinelli.
Carey, B. (2005a). 'Snake Phobias, Moodiness and a Battle in Psychiatry'. *New York Times*, 18 June 2005.
—— (2005b). 'Who's Mentally Ill? Deciding Is Often All in the Mind'. *New York Times*, 12 June.
Carothers, A. (1954). *Normal and Pathological Psychology of the African: Ethnopsychiatric Studies*. Paris: Masson.
Carver, C.S., and Miller, C.J. (2006). 'Relations of Serotonin Function to Personality: Current Views and a Key Methodological Issue'. *Psychiatry Research*, 144, pp. 1–15.
Castel, R. (1973). *Le Psychanalysme: L'ordre psychanalytique et le pouvoir*. Paris: Maspero.
—— (1978). *Lo psicoanalismo*. Translated by L. Fontana. Turin: Einaudi.
—— (1992). 'Two Readings of *Histoire de la Folie* in France'. In: Still, A., and Velody, I. (eds), *Rewriting the History of Madness*. London: Routledge, pp. 65–68.
—— (2005). 'Michel Foucault e le critiche della psichiatria: una lettura soggettiva'. *Rivista Sperimentale di Freniatria*, CXXIV(3 sup.).
Chiesa, L. (2011). 'The Bio-Theo-Politics of Birth'. *Angelaki*, 16 (3), pp. 101–15.
Civita, A. (1999). 'La clinica moderna e la malattia mentale'. In: Civita, A. and Cosenza, D. (eds), *La cura della malattia mentale. Vol. 1. Storia ed Epistemologia*. Milan: Bruno Mondadori, pp. 89–133.

Colucci, M. (1998). 'Il vetro dell'acquario. Michel Foucault e le istituzioni della psichiatria'. *aut aut*, 285–86, pp. 69–86.
—— (2004). 'Isterici, internati, uomini infami: Michel Foucault e la resistenza al potere'. *aut aut*, 323, pp. 97–110.
—— (2006a). 'Foucault and Psychiatric Power After *Madness and Civilization*'. In: Beaulieu, A., and Gabbard, D. (eds), *Michel Foucault and Power Today: International Multidisciplinary Studies in the History of the Present*. Oxford: Lexington Books, pp. 61–70.
—— (2006b). 'Medicalizzazione'. In: *Lessico di biopolitca*. Rome: Manifesto Libri, pp. 175–81.
—— (2008). 'Scienza del pericolo, clinica del deficit: Sulla medicalizzazione in psichiatria'. *aut aut*, 340, pp. 105–22.
Colucci, M. and Di Vittorio, P. (2001). *Franco Basaglia*, Milan: Mondadori Bruno.
Cook, D. (1990). 'Madness and the Cogito: Derrida's Critique of *Folie et Déraison*'. *Journal of the British Society for Phenomenology*, 21(2), pp. 164–74.
Cooper, D.G. (1967). *Psychiatry and Anti-Psychiatry*. London: Travistock.
Cooper, D.G., et al. (1988). 'Confinement, Psychiatry, Prison'. In: Kritzman, L.D. (ed.), *Politics, Philosophy, Culture: Interviews and Other Writings, 1977–1984*, Vol. 3. London: Routledge, 2004, pp. 178–226.
Corbellini, G. and Jervis, G. (2008). *La razionalità negata: Psichiatria e antipsichiatria in Italia*. Turin: Bollati Boringhieri.
Crossley, N. (1999). 'Working Utopias and Social Movements: An Investigation Using Case Study Materials from Radical Mental Health Movements in Britain'. *Sociology*, 33(4), pp. 809–30.
—— (2006). *Contesting Psychiatry: Social Movements in Mental Health*. London: Routledge.
Crow, T.J. (1980). 'Molecular Pathology of Schizophrenia: More Than One Disease Process?' *British Medical Journal*, 280, pp. 66–68.
—— (1986). 'The Continuum of Psychosis and its Implication for the Structure of the Gene'. *British Journal of Psychiatry*, 149, pp. 419–29.
—— (1990). 'Temporal Lobe Asymmetries as the Key to the Etiology of Schizophrenia'. *Schizophrenia Bulletin*, 16, pp. 433–44.
Curtis, B. (2002). 'Foucault on Governamentality and Population: The Impossible Discovery'. *Canadian Journal of Sociology*, 27(4), pp. 505–33.
Curto, A. (2005). 'Introduzione. Che cosa significa "biopolitica"?'. In: Curto, A. (ed.), *Biopolitica: Storia e attualità di un concetto*. Verona: Ombre Corte, pp. 7–43.
D'Amico, R. (1984). 'Text and Context: Derrida and Foucault on Descartes'. In: Fekete, J. (ed.), *The Structural Allegory: Reconstructive Encounters with the New French Thought*. Minneapolis: University of Minnesota Press, pp. 164–82.

Daumezon, G., and Koechlin, P. (1952). 'Psychothérapie française institutionnelle contemporaine'. *Anais portugeses de psiquiatria*, Vol. 4, pp. 271–312.
Davydov, J.U. (1966). *Il lavoro e la libertà*. Turin: Einaudi.
Dain, N. (1989). 'Critics and Dissenters: Reflections on Anti-psychiatry in the United States'. *Journal of the History of the Behavioral Sciences*, 25(1), pp. 3–25.
De Giorgi, A. (2006). 'Discipline'. In: *Lessico di Biopolitica*. Rome: Manifesto Libri, pp. 119–23.
De Girolamo, G., et al. (2007). 'The Current State of Mental Health Care in Italy: Problems, Perspectives, and Lessons to Learn'. *European Archives of Psychiatry and Clinical Neurosciences*, 257, pp. 83–91.
De Peri, F. (1984). 'Il medico e il folle: Istituzione psichiatrica, sapere scientifico e pensiero medico fra Otto e Novecento'. In: Della Peruta, F. (ed.), *Storia d'Italia, Annali 7, Malati e medicina*. Turin: Einaudi.
Dell'Acqua, G. (2008a). 'Il Miraggio Del Farmaco'. *aut aut*, 340, pp. 93–104.
—— (2008b). 'Il parere di Dell'Acqua'. Available at <http://news2000.libero.it/speciali/sp63/pg4.html>, accessed 19 December 2008.
Dell'Acqua, G., and Camarlinghi, R. (2008). 'Le scommesse di Basaglia: Intervista a Peppe Dell'Acqua a cura di Roberto Camarlinghi'. *Animazione Sociale*, 219(1), pp. 3–14.
Derrida, J. (2001). 'Cogito and the History of Madness'. Translated by Alan Bass. In: Derrida, J., *Writing and Difference*. London: Routledge, pp. 36–76.
Descartes, R. (1985). 'First Meditation'. Translated by John Cottingham, Robert Stoothoff and Dugald Murdoch, in: *The Philosophical Writings of Descartes*, Vol. II. Cambridge: Cambridge University Press.
Di Fusco, C., and Kirchmayr, R. (1995). 'Secondo seminario: Quale corpo? – discussione'. In: Laboratorio di Filosofia Contemporanea, *Follia e Paradosso. Seminari sul pensiero di Basaglia*.Trieste: Edizioni E, pp. 75–85.
Di Vittorio, P. (1999). *Foucault e Basaglia: L'incontro tra genealogie e movimenti di base*. Verona: Ombre Corte.
—— (2004a). 'Biopolitica e psichiatria'. *aut aut*, 323, pp. 159–74.
—— (2006). 'From Psychiatry to Bio-Politics or the Birth of the Bio-Security State'. In: Beaulieu, A., and Gabbard, D. (eds), *Michel Foucault and Power Today: International Multidisciplinary Studies in the History of the Present*. Oxford: Lexington Books, pp. 71–80.
Dilthey, W. (1976). 'Ideas about a Descriptive and Analytical Psychology'. In: Rickman, H.P. (ed.), *Selected Writings*. Cambridge: Cambridge University Press, pp. 87–97.
—— (1989). *Introduction to the Human Sciences*. Princeton: Princeton University Press.
Donnelly, M. (1992). *The Politics of Mental Health in Italy*. London: Routledge.

Dreyfus, H.L. (1987). 'Foreword to the California Edition'. In: *Mental Illness and Psychology*. Berkeley: University of California Press, pp. vii–xliii.

Dreyfus, H.L., and Rabinow, P. (1982). *Michel Foucault: Beyond Structuralism and Hermeneutics*. Brighton: Harvester.

Elden, S. (2006). *Discipline, Health and Madness: Foucault's 'Le Pouvoir psychiatrique'*. London: SAGE.

Eng, E.W. (1968). 'Body, We-awareness, and Therapeutic Community'. *Psychotherapy and Psychosomatics*, 16, pp. 183–88.

Engel, G. (1977). 'The Need for a New Medical Model: a Challenge for Biomedicine'. *Science* 196(4286): 129–36.

Esposito, R. (1998). *Communitas. Origine e destino della comunità*. Turin: Einaudi.

—— (2002). *Immunitas. Protezione e negazione della vita*. Turin: Einaudi.

—— (2004). *Bíos. Biopolitica e filosofia*. Turin: Einaudi.

—— (2005). 'Biopolitica, immunità, comunità'. In: Cutro, A. (ed.), *Biopolitica: Storia ed attualità di un concetto*. Verona: Ombre Corte, pp. 158–67.

—— (2007). *Terza persona: Politica della vita e filosofia dell'impersonale*. Turin: Einaudi.

—— (2008a). 'Prefazione'. In: Bazzicalupo, L. (ed.), *Impersonale: In dialogo con Roberto Esposito*. Milan and Udine: Mimesis, pp. 9–39.

—— (2008b). *Termini della politica: Comunità, immunità, biopolitica*. Milan and Udine: Mimesis.

Fanon, F. (1961). *The Wretched of the Earth*. Translated by Richard Philcox. London: Penguin.

Fennell, P. (1996). *Treatment Without Consent: Law, Psychiatry and the Treatment of Mentally Disordered People Since 1845*. London: Routledge.

First, M.B. (2005). 'Mutually Exclusive Versus Co-occurring Diagnostic Categories: The Challenge of Diagnostic Comorbidity'. *Psychopathology*, 38, pp. 206–10.

Flaherty, P. (1986). '(Con)textual Contest: Derrida and Foucault on Madness and the Cartesian Subject'. *Philosophy of the Social Sciences* 16(1), pp. 157–75.

Foucault, M. (1954). *Maladie mentale et personnalité*. Paris: PUF.

—— (1962). *Maladie mentale et psychologie*. Paris: PUF.

—— (1976a). 'Crisis de un modelo en la medicina?' *Revista centroamericana de ciencias de la salud*, 3, pp. 197–209.

—— (1976b). 'La crisis de la medicina o la crisis de la antimedicina'. *Educación Médica y Salud*, 10, pp. 152–70.

—— (1977). *Microfisica del potere: Interventi politici*, ed. Fontana, A. and Pasquino, P. Turin: Einaudi.

—— (1978). *I, Pierre Rivière, having slaughtered my mother, my sister and my brother: A Case of Parricide in the 19th Century*. Translated by Frank Jellinek. London: Penguin.

—— (1982). 'The Subject and Power'. In: Foucault, M., *Michel Foucault: Beyond Structuralism and Hermeneutics*, ed. Dreyfus, H.L. and Rabinow, P. Brighton: Harvester, pp. 208–26.
—— (1984a). 'Preface to the History of Sexuality, Volume II'. Translated by William Smock. In: Foucault, M., *The Foucault Reader*, ed. Rabinow, P. New York: Pantheon Books, pp. 333–39.
—— (1984b). 'Dream, Imagination, and Existence'. Translated by Forrest Williams, *Review of Existential Psychology and Psychiatry*, XIX(1) 1984–85, pp. 29–78.
—— (1986). 'Truth and Power'. In: Foucault, M., *The Foucault Reader*, Rabinow, P. (ed.). London: Penguin, pp. 51–75.
—— (1987). *Mental Illness and Psychology*. Translated by Alan Sheridan. Berkeley: University of California Press.
—— (1988). 'Technologies of the Self'. In: Foucault, M., *Technologies of the Self: A Seminar With Michel Foucault*, ed. Martin, L.H., Gutman, H., and Hutton, P.H. London: Tavistock, pp. 16–49.
—— (1991). *Discipline and Punish: The Birth of the Prison*. Translated by Alan Sheridan. London: Penguin.
—— (1994a). 'Crisis de un modelo en la medicina?' In: *Dits et Ecrits*, Vol. 3. Paris: Gallimard, pp. 40–58.
—— (1994b). 'Folie, une question de pouvoir'. In: *Dits et écrits*, Vol. 2. Paris: Gallimard, pp. 660–64.
—— (1994c). 'L'asile illimité'. In: *Dits et écrits*, Vol. 3. Paris: Gallimard, pp. 271–75.
—— (1994d). 'Un problème m'interésse depuis longtemps, c'est celui du système pénal'. In: *Dits et Écrits*, Vol. 2. Paris: Gallimard, pp. 205–10.
—— (1997a). 'Crisi della medicina o crisi dell'antimedicina?' In: Foucault, M., *Archivio Foucault*, ed. Dal Lago, A., Vol. 2. Milan: Feltrinelli, pp. 202–19.
—— (1997b). 'Technologies of the Self'. In: Foucault, M., *Ethics: Subjectivity and Truth*, ed. Rabinow, P. New York: The New Press, pp. 232–52.
—— (1998). *The History of Sexuality: 1. The Will to Knowledge*. Translated by Robert Hurley. London: Penguin.
—— (2001). *Madness and Civilization: A History of Insanity in the Age of Reason*. Translated by Richard Howard. London: Routledge.
—— (2002a). 'First Preface to Histoire de la folie à l'âge classique (1961)'. *Pli, The Warwick Journal of Philosophy*, 13, pp. 1–10.
—— (2002b). *The Archeology of Knowledge*. Translated by Alan Sheridan. London: Routledge.
—— (2003a). *Abnormal: Lectures at the Collège de France, 1974–1975*. Translated by Graham Burchell. New York: Picador.

—— (2003b). *Society Must Be Defended: Lectures at the Collège de France, 1975–1976*. Translated by David Macey. New York: Picador.

—— (2004). 'The Crisis of Medicine or the Crisis of Antimedicine?' *Foucault Studies*, 1, pp. 5–19.

—— (2005). *The Hermeneutics of the Subject: Lectures at the Collège de France, 1981–1982*. Translated by Graham Burchell. New York: Picador.

—— (2006a). *History of Madness*. Translated by Jonathan Murphy and Jean Khalfa. London: Routledge.

—— (2006b). *Psychiatric Power: Lectures at the Collège de France, 1973–1974*. Translated by Graham Burchell. New York: Palgrave Macmillan.

—— (2008a). *The Birth of the Clinic: An Archaeology of Medical Perception*. Translated by Alan Sheridan. London: Routledge.

—— (2008b). *The Birth of Biopolitics: Lectures at the Collège de France, 1978–1979*. Translated by Graham Burchell. New York: Palgrave Macmillan.

Foucault, M. and Ruas, C. (2004). 'An Interview With Michel Foucault'. In: *Death and the Labyrinth*. London: Continuum, pp. 171–88.

Foucault, M., and Trombadori, D. (2001). 'Interview with Michel Foucault'. In: Foucault, M., *The Essential Works of Foucault, 1954–1984, Volume 3: Power*, ed. Faubion, James D. New York: New Press, pp. 239–97.

Foucault, M., et al. (1994). 'Table ronde sur l'expertise psychiatrique'. In: *Dits et écrits*, Vol.2, Paris: Gallimard, pp. 664–74.

Freud, S. (1901). *The Psychopathology of Everyday Life*. Translated by James Strachey. In: *The Standard Edition of the Complete Psychological Works of Sigmund Freud*, Vol. 6. London: Hogarth Press and Institute of Psycho-Analysis.

—— (1923). 'Two Encyclopaedia Articles: Psychoanalysis and the Libido Theory'. Translated by James Strachey. In: *The Standard Edition of the Complete Psychological Works of Sigmund Freud*, Vol. 18. London: Hogarth Press and Institute of Psycho-Analysis, pp. 233–59.

—— (1924). 'Neurosis and Psychosis'. Translated by James Strachey. In: *The Standard Edition of the Complete Psychological Works of Sigmund Freud*, Vol. 19. London: Hogarth Press and Institute of Psycho-Analysis, pp. 147–53.

Freud, S., and Binswanger, L. (2000). *The Freud-Binswanger Letters*. Translated by Tom Roberts and Arnold Pomerans. London: Open Gate Press.

Freud, S., and Breuer, J. (1895). 'Studies in Hysteria'. Translated by James Strachey. In: *The Standard Edition of the Complete Psychological Works of Sigmund Freud*, Vol. 2. London: Hogarth Press and Institute of Psycho-Analysis, pp. 48–106.

Galimberti, U. (2005). *La casa di psiche. Dalla psicoanalisi alla pratica filosofica*. Milan: Feltrinelli.

—— (2007). *Psichiatria e fenomenologia*. Milan: Feltrinelli.

Gallio, G. (2009a). 'Le riunioni di Colorno. Introduzione ai verbali'. *aut aut*, 342, pp. 48–67.
—— (ed.) (2009b). *Basaglia a Colorno, aut aut* 342, April–June 2009. Milan: Il Saggiatore.
Galzigna, M. (2006). *Il mondo nella mente. Per un'epistemologia della cura.* Venice: Marsilio.
Gambescia, C. (2010). 'Prefazione'. In: *Oltre l'utopia basagliana. Per un nuovo paradigma della psichiatria.* Milan and Udine: Mimesis, pp. 13–18.
Gershman, C. (1984). 'Psychiatric abuse in the Soviet Union'. *Society*, 21(5), pp. 54–59.
Giannichedda, M.G. (2005). 'Introduzione'. In: Ongaro Basaglia, F. (ed.), *L'utopia della realtà.* Turin: Einaudi, pp. vii–lii.
—— (2009). 'Intervento al corso universitario specialistico "Il pensiero di Franco Basaglia"'. [lecture] (14 January 2009).
Girone, E. (1953). *Io e i pazzi.* Milan: Ceschini.
Goffman, E. (2007). *Asylums: Essays on the Social Situation of Mental Patients and Other Inmates.* New Brunswick: Transaction.
Goldberg, D., and Goodyer, I. (2005). *The Origins and Course of Common Mental Disorders.* London: Taylor and Francis.
Goldberg, D. and Huxley, P.J. (1980). *Mental Illness in the Community: The Pathway to Psychiatric Care.* London: Tavistock.
Gramsci, A. (1977). *Quaderni del carcere. Volume Terzo. Quaderni 12–29.* Turin: Einaudi.
Griesinger, W. (1965). *Mental Pathology and Therapeutics.* Translated by Lockhart Robertson and James Rutherford. New York: Hafner.
Gruppo Nazionale PROGRES (2001). 'Le strutture residenziali psichiatriche in Italia: risultati della fase 1 del progetto PROGRES'. *Epidemiologia e Psichiatria Sociale*, 10, pp. 260–75.
Gutting, G. (2005). 'Foucault and the History of Madness'. In: Gutting, G. (ed.), *The Cambridge Companion to Foucault.* Cambridge: Cambridge University Press, pp. 47–70.
Hacking, I. (1986). 'The Archaeology of Foucault'. In: Hoy, D. (ed.), *Foucault: A Critical Reader.* Oxford: Blackwell, pp. 27–40.
Häfner, H. (1961). *Psychopathen.* Berlin: Springer.
Harrington, M., et al. (2002). 'The Results of a Multi-Centre Audit of the Prescribing of Antipsychotic Drugs for In-patients in the UK'. *Psychiatric Bulletin*, 26, pp. 414–18.
Hartmann, H. (1964). *Essays on Ego Psychology.* New York: International University Press.
Healy, D. (1997). *The Antidepressant Era.* Cambridge, MA: Harvard University Press.

—— (2002). *The Creation of Psychopharmacology*. Cambridge, MA: Harvard University Press.
Heidegger, M. (1967). *Being and Time*. Translated by John Macquarrie and Edward Robinson. Oxford: Blackwell.
Holmer Nadesan, M. (2008). *Governamentality, Biopower and Everyday Life*. London: Routledge.
Hopton, J. (1995). 'The Application of the Ideas of Frantz Fanon to the Practice of Mental Health Nursing'. *Journal of Advanced Nursing*, 21(4), pp. 723–28.
Husserl, E. (1931). *Ideas: General Introduction to Pure Phenomenology*. Translated by W.R. Boyce Gibson. London: Macmillan.
—— (1970). *Crisis of the European Sciences and Transcendental Phenomenology: An Introduction to Phenomenological Philosophy*. Translated by David Carr. Evanston: Northwestern University Press.
INSERM (2004). 'Psychotherapie: trois approches évaluées'. In: INSERM (ed.), *Expertise Collective*. Paris: INSERM.
ISTAT (2008). 'L'ospedalizzazione dei pazienti affetti da disturbi psichici'. Available at <http://www.istat.it/dati/dataset/20080401_01/notainformativa.pdf>, accessed 13 March 2010.
Jacobi, F., et al. (2004). 'Prevalence, Co-morbidity and Correlates of Mental Disorders in the General Population: Results from the German Health Interview and Examination Survey (GHS)'. *Psychological Medicine*, 34(4), pp. 597–611.
Jacobson, E. (1972). *Depression: Comparative Studies of Normal, Neurotic, and Psychotic Conditions*. New York: International University Press.
Jansen, E. (1980). 'Editor's Discussion'. In: Jansen, E. (ed.), *The Therapeutic Community: Outside the Hospital*. London: Richmond Fellowship, pp. 19–51.
Jaspers, K. (1963). *General Psychopathology*. Translated by J. Hoenig and M. Hamilton. Chicago: University of Chicago Press.
Jervis, G. (1975). *Manuale critico di psichiatria*. Milan: Feltrinelli.
Jones, M. (1968). *Beyond the Therapeutic Community: Social Learning and Social Psychiatry*. New Haven and London: Yale University Press.
Kaiser, S. (1990). *The Social Psychology of Clothing: Symbolic Appearances in Context*. London: Macmillan.
Katschnig, H., and Windhaber, J. (1998). 'Die Kombination einer Neuroleptika-Langzeitmedikation mit psychosozialen Massnahmen'. In: Riederer, P., Laux, G., and Pöldinger, W. (eds), *Neuro-Psychopharmaka – Ein Therapie-Handbuch. Band 4: Neuroleptika. 2. Auflage*. Vienna: Springer-Verlag.
Kazdin, A.E. (1996). *Conduct Disorders in Childhood and Adolescence*. London: SAGE.
Kernberg, O.F. (1975). *Borderline Conditions and Pathological Narcissism*. New York: Jason Aronson.

Kessler, R.C. et al. (1994). 'Lifetime and 12-Month Prevalence of DSM-III-R Psychiatric Disorders in the United States: Results from the National Comorbidity Survey', *Archives of General Psychiatry*, 51(1), pp. 8–19.

—— et al. (2005). 'Prevalence, Severity, and Comorbidity of 12-month DSM–IV Disorders in the National Comorbidity Survey Replication'. *Archives of General Psychiatry*, 62, pp. 617–27.

Khalfa, J. (2006). 'Introduction'. In: *History of Madness*. London: Routledge, pp. xiii–xxv.

Kimura, B. (1982). 'The Phenomenology of the Between: The Problem of the Basic Disturbance of Schizophrenia'. In: De Koning, A.J.J., and Jenner, F.A. (eds), *Phenomenology and Psychiatry*. London: Grune and Stratton, pp. 173–85.

Kjellen, R. (1920). *Grundriß zu einem System der Politik*. Leipzig: S. Hirzel Verlag.

Knapp, M., et al. (2007). 'Mental Health Policy and Practice Across Europe: an Overview'. In: Knapp, M., McDaid, D., Mossialoss, E., and Thornicroft, G. (eds), *Mental Health Policy and Practice Across Europe: The Future Direction of Mental Health Care*. New York: Open University Press, pp. 1–14.

Kramer, P.D. (1993). *Listening to Prozac*. London: Penguin Books.

Laboratorio di Filosofia Contemporanea (ed.) (1995). *Follia e paradosso. Seminari sul pensiero di Basaglia*. Trieste: Edizioni E.

LaCapra, D. (1990). 'Foucault, History, and Madness'. *History of the Human Sciences*, 3(1), pp. 31–38.

Laing, A. (1997). *R.D. Laing and the Paths of Anti-Psychiatry*. London: Routledge.

Laing, R.D. (1964). 'What is Schizophrenia?' *New Left Review* 28 (Nov.–Dec. 1964), pp. 63–68.

—— (1990). *The Divided Self*. London: Penguin.

Law, J. (2006). *Big Pharma: Exposing the Global Healthcare Agenda*. New York: Carroll and Graf.

Lehtinen, V., et al. (2007). 'Developments in the Treatment of Mental Disorders'. In: Knapp, M., McDaid, D., Mossialoss, E., and Thornicroft, G. (eds), *Mental Health Policy and Practice Across Europe: The Future Direction of Mental Health Care*. New York: Open University Press, pp. 126–45.

Lemke, T. (2011). *Biopolitics: An Advanced Introduction*. Translated by Erik Frederik Trump. New York: New York University Press.

Leoni, F. (ed.) (2011). *Franco Basaglia: Un laboratorio italiano*. Milan: Bruno Mondadori.

Lombroso, C. (1896). *L'uomo delinquente in rapporto all'antropologia, alla giurisprudenza ed alle discipline carcerarie*. Turin: Fratelli Bocca.

Lovell, A.M., and Scheper-Hughes, N. (1987). 'Introduction. The Utopia of Reality: Franco Basaglia and the Practice of a Democratic Psychiatry'. In: Scheper-Hughes,

N., and Lovell, A.M. (eds), *Psychiatry Inside Out: Selected Writings of Franco Basaglia*. New York: Columbia University Press, pp. 1–50.

Magliano, L., et al. (2002). 'The Impact of Professional and Social Support on the Burden of Families of Patients with Schizophrenia in Italy'. *Acta Psychiatrica Scandinava*, 106, pp. 291–98.

Main, T. (1946). 'The Hospital as a Therapeutic Institution'. *Bulletin of the Menninger Clinic*, 10, pp. 66–70.

Mannheim, K. (1936). *Ideology and Utopia: An Introduction to the Sociology of Knowledge*. London and New York: Brace and Company.

Maone, A., et al. (2002). 'Day Programs in Italy for Persons with Severe Mental Illness: A Nationwide Survey'. *International Journal of Mental Health*, 31, pp. 30–49.

Marder, S.R., et al. (2003). 'Maintenance Treatment of Schizophrenia with Risperidone or Haloperidol: 2-Year Outcomes'. *American Journal of Psychiatry*, 160(8), pp. 1405–12.

Marx, K., and Engels, F. (1970). *The German Ideology*. Translated by C.J. Arthur. London: Lawrence and Wishart.

Massi, A. (ed.) (2010). Franco Basaglia e la filosofia del '900. Milan: Bema.

May, T. (2006). 'Foucault's Relation to Phenomenology'. In: Gutting, G. (ed.), *The Cambridge Companion to Foucault*. Cambridge: Cambridge University Press.

McCall, R.J. (1983). *Phenomenological Psychology: An Introduction*. Madison: University of Wisconsin Press.

Meloni, M. (2011). 'Naturalism as an Ontology of Ourselves'. *Telos*, 155, pp. 151–74.

Meltzer, H., et al. (1995). *The Prevalence of Psychiatric Morbidity Among Adults Living in Private Households: OPCS Surveys of Psychiatric Morbidity in Great Britain. Report 1*. London: HMSO.

Mental Disability Advocacy Center (2005). *The Right to Vote at Risk in Bulgaria*. Budapest: Mental Disability Advocacy Center.

Merleau-Ponty, M. (2002). *Phenomenology of Perception*. Translated by Colin Smith. London: Routledge.

Midelfort, E.H.C. (1980). 'Madness and Civilization in Early Modern Europe: A Reappraisal of Michel Foucault'. In: Malament, B. (ed.), *After the Reformation: Essays in Honor of J.H. Hexter*. Philadelphia: University of Pennsylvania Press, pp. 247–66.

Mills, J.A., and Harrison, T. (2007). 'John Rickman, Wilfred Ruprecht Bion, and the Origins of the Therapeutic Community'. *History of Psychology*, 10(1), pp. 22–43.

Minkowski, E. (1970). *Lived Time. Phenomenological and Psychopathological Studies*. Translated by Nancy Metzel. Evanston: Northwestern University Press.

Mollica, R.F. (1985). 'The Unfinished Revolution in Italian Psychiatry: An International Perspective'. *International Journal of Mental Health*, 14(1–2).

Moncrieff, J., and Cohen, D. (2005). 'Rethinking Models of Psychotropic Drug Action'. *Psychotherapy and Psychosomatics*, 74, pp. 145–53.

Morlino, M., et al. (1993). 'Interventi psicoterapici nei Dipartimenti di Salute Mentale di Napoli: un'indagine sulle scelte e sulla qualificazione degli operatori'. *Epidemiologia e Psichiatria Sociale*, 2, pp. 25–34.

Munizza, C., et al. (1995). 'Prescription Pattern of Antidepressants in Out-Patient Psychiatric Practice'. *Psychological Medicine*, 25, pp. 771–78.

Murray, C., and Lopez, A. (1996). *The Global Burden of Disease*. Cambridge, MA: Harvard University Press.

Ongaro Basaglia, F. (1987). 'Preface'. In: Scheper-Hughes, N., and Lovell, A.M. (eds), *Psychiatry Inside Out: Selected Writings of Franco Basaglia*. New York: Columbia University Press, pp. xi–xxvi.

—— (1998). 'I vent'anni della legge 180. Il primato della pratica in psichiatria'. Available at <http://www.psychiatryonline.it/ital/180/ongaro2.htm>, accessed 12 March 2010.

Paris, J. (2008). *Prescriptions for the Mind: A Critical View of Contemporary Psychiatry*. Oxford: Oxford University Press.

Parmegiani, F., and Zanetti, M. (2007). *Basaglia, una biografia*. Trieste: Lint.

Phillips, J. (2004). 'Understanding/Explanation'. In: Radden, J. (ed.), *The Philosophy of Psychiatry*. Oxford: Oxford University Press, pp. 180–90.

Picardi, A., et al. (2003). 'Le strutture residenziali psichiatriche in Italia. Risultati preliminari della fase 2 del progetto PROGRES'. *Notiziario dell'Istituto Superiore di Sanità*, pp. 3–9.

Piccione, R. (2004). *Il futuro dei servizi di salute mentale in Italia. Significato e prospettive del sistema italiano di promozione e protezione della salute mentale*. Milan: Franco Angeli.

Pinel, P. (1806). *Treatise on Insanity*. Translated by D.D. Davis. Sheffield: W. Todd.

Pirella, A. (1987). 'Institutional Psychiatry Between Transformation and Rationalization: The Case of Italy'. *International Journal of Mental Health*, 16(1–2), pp. 118–41.

Pirkola, S. et al. (2005). 'DSM–IV Mood, Anxiety and Alcohol Use Disorders and Their Comorbidity in the Finnish General Population: Results from the Health 2000 Study'. *Social Psychiatry and Psychiatric Epidemiology*, 40(1), pp. 1–10.

Pitrelli, N. (2004). *L'uomo che restituì la parola ai matti: Franco Basaglia, la comunicazione e la fine dei manicomi*. Naples: Editori Riuniti.

Pivetta, O. (2012). *Franco Basaglia, il dottore dei matti: La biografia*. Milan: Dalai.

Pizza, G. (2007). 'La questione corporea nell'opera di Franco Basaglia: Note antropologiche'. *Rivista sperimentale di freniatria*, CXXXI(1), pp. 49–67.

Priebe, S. et al. (2005). 'Reinstitutionalization in Mental Health Care: Comparison of Data on Service Provision from Six European Countries'. *British Medical Journal*, 330(7483), 123–26.
Rabinow, P., and Rose, N. (2006). 'Biopower Today'. *Biosciences*, 1(2), pp. 195–217.
Read, J., and Bentall, R. (2010). 'The Effectiveness of Electroconvulsive Therapy: A Literature Review'. *Epidemiologia e psichiatria sociale*, 19(4), pp. 333–47.
Richter, D. (1971). 'Political Dissenters in Mental Hospitals'. *The British Journal of Psychiatry*, 119(549), pp. 225–26.
Rigier, D. (2007). 'Dimensional Approaches to Psychiatric Classification: Refining the Research Agenda for DSM–V: An Introduction'. *International Journal of Methods in Psychiatric Research.* 16(S1): S1–S5.
Roberts, M. (2005). 'The Production of the Psychiatric Subject: Power, Knowledge and Michel Foucault'. *Nursing Philosophy*, 6, pp. 33–46.
Rose, N. (1999). 'Medicine, History and the Present'. In: *Reassessing Foucault: Power, Medicine and the Body*. London: Routledge, pp. 48–72.
—— (2001). 'The Politics of Life Itself'. *Theory, Culture and Society*, 18, pp. 1–30.
—— (2003). 'Neurochemical Selves'. *Society*, 41, pp. 46–59.
—— (2007a). *The Politics of Life Itself: Biomedicine, Power, and Subjectivity in the Twenty-First Century.* Princeton: Princeton University Press.
—— (2007b). 'Psychopharmaceuticals in Europe'. In: Knapp, M., McDaid, D., Mossialoss, E., and Thornicroft, G. (eds), *Mental Health Policy and Practice Across Europe: The Future Direction of Mental Health Care*. New York: Open University Press, pp. 146–87.
Rose, N., and Novas, C. (2004). 'Biological Citizenship'. In: Ong, A., and Collier, S. (eds), *Global Assemblages: Technology, Politics, and Ethics as Anthropological Problems*, Oxford: Blackwell, pp. 439–63.
Rotelli, F. (1994). *Per la normalità. Taccuino di uno psichiatra*. Trieste: Asterios.
—— (1999). 'Quale politica per la salute mentale alla fine di un secolo di riforme?' *La psicoanalisi*, 25, pp. 92–99.
—— (2005). 'Foucault a Trieste'. *Rivista sperimentale di freniatria*, 3(S), pp. 36–39.
Roth, A., and Fonagy, P. (2004). *What Works for Whom: A Critical Review of Psychotherapy Research*. New York: The Guilford Press.
Rouse, J. (2005). 'Power/Knowledge'. In: Gutting, G. (ed.), *The Cambridge Companion to Foucault*. Cambridge: Cambridge University Press, pp. 95–122.
Rovatti, P.A. (1995). 'Cosa possiamo scrivere nel piccolo libro?' In: Laboratorio di Filosofia Contemporanea (ed.), *Follia e paradosso. Seminari sul pensiero di Basaglia*. Trieste: Edizioni E, pp. 127–32.
—— (2008). 'Il soggetto che non c'è'. In: Galzigna, M. (ed.), *Foucault, Oggi*. Milan: Feltrinelli, pp. 216–25.

Sartre, J.-P. (1948). *Situations II*. Paris: Gallimard.
—— (1975). *Between Existentialism and Marxism*. Translated by John Matthews. New York: Verso Books.
——(1978). *Being and Nothingness; an Essay on Phenomenological Ontology*. Translated by Hazel E. Barnes. New York: Pocket Books.
Sayce, L., and Curran, C. (2007). 'Tackling Social Exclusion Across Europe'. In: Knapp, M., McDaid, D., Mossialoss, E., and Thornicroft, G. (eds), *Mental Health Policy and Practice Across Europe: The Future Direction of Mental Health Care*. New York: Open University Press, pp. 34–59.
Schatzberg, A. and Nemeroff, C. (2004). *The American Psychiatric Publishing Textbook of Psychopharmacology* (3rd edn). Washington, DC: American Psychiatric Press.
Schoevers, R.A., et al. (2006). 'Prevention of Late-Life Depression in Primary Care: Do We Know Where to Begin?' *American Journal of Psychiatry*, 163, pp. 1611–21.
Scull, A. (1990). 'Michel Foucault's History of Madness'. *History of the Human Sciences*, 3(1), pp. 57–67.
Sedgwick, P. (1982). *Psycho Politics*. London: Pluto Press Limited.
Segatori, A. (2010). *Oltre l'utopia basagliana. Per un nuovo paradigma della psichiatria*. Milan and Udine: Mimesis.
Seigel, J. (1990). 'Avoiding the Subject: A Foucaultian Itinerary'. *Journal of the History of Ideas*, 51(20), pp. 273–99.
Shorter, E. (1997). *A History of Psychiatry: From the Era of the Asylum to the Age of Prozac*. New York: John Wiley and Sons.
Sigerist, H.E. (1932). *Man and Medicine: An Introduction to Medical Knowledge*. Translated by Margaret Gal Boise. London: W.W. Norton and Co.
Singh, I., and Rose, N. (2009). 'Biomarkers in Psychiatry'. *Nature*, 460 (9 July), pp. 202–7.
Smith, C. (2000). 'The Sovereign State v. Foucault: Law and Disciplinary Power'. *The Sociological Review*, 48(2), pp. 283–306.
Social Exclusion Unit (2004). *Mental Health and Social Exclusion*. London: Office of the Deputy Prime Minister.
Spiegelberg, H. (1972). *Phenomenology in Psychology and Psychiatry: A Historical Introduction*. Evanston: Northwestern University Press.
Stiles, W.B., et al. (2006). 'Effectiveness of Cognitive-Behavioural, Person-Centred and Psychodynamic Therapies as Practised in UK National Health Service Settings'. *Psychological Medicine*, 36(4), pp. 555–66.
Still, A., and Velody, I. (1992). 'Introduction'. In: Still, A. and Velody, I. (eds), *Rewriting the History of Madness*. London: Routledge, pp. 1–16.
Stoppa, F. (2006). *La prima curva dopo il paradiso. Per una poetica del lavoro nelle istituzioni*. Rome: Borla.
Szasz, T.S. (1960). 'The Myth of Mental Illness'. *American Psychologist*, 15, pp. 113–18.

—— (2003). *The Myth of Mental Illness. Foundations of a Theory of Personal Conduct*. New York: Perennial.
Tansella, M., and Thornicroft, G. (2000). 'Planning and Providing Mental Health Services for a Community'. In: Gelder, M., Andreasen, N., Lopez-Ibor, J., and Geddes, J. (eds), *New Oxford Textbook of Psychiatry*, Vol. 2. Oxford: Oxford University Press, pp. 1547–58.
Tarizzo, D. (2011). 'Biopolitics and the Ideology of "Mental Health"'. *Filozofski vestnik*, XXXII(2), pp. 135–49.
Thornicroft, G. (2006). *Shunned: Discrimination against People with Mental Illness*. Oxford: Oxford University Press.
Tibaldi, G., et al. (1997). 'Utilization of Neuroleptic Drugs in Italian Mental Health Services: A Survey in Piedmont'. *Psychiatric Services*, 48, pp. 213–17.
Tognoni, G. (1999). 'Pharmacoepidemiology of Psychotropic Drugs in Patients with Severe Mental Disorders in Italy: Italian Collaborative Study Group on the Outcome of Severe Mental Disorders'. *European Journal of Clinical Pharmacology*, 55, pp. 685–60.
Tomasi, R., et al. (2006). 'The Prescription of Psychotropic Drugs in Psychiatric Residential Facilities: A National Survey in Italy'. *Acta Psychiatrica Scandinava*, 113, pp. 212–23.
Tomov, T., et al. (2007). 'Mental Health Policy in Former Eastern Bloc Countries'. In: Knapp, M., McDaid, D., Mossialoss, E., and Thornicroft, G. (eds), *Mental Health Policy and Practice Across Europe: The Future Direction of Mental Health Care*. New York: Open University Press, pp. 397–425.
Valenstein, E. (1998). *Blaming the Brain: The Truth About Drugs and Mental Illness*. New York: The Free Press.
Vedantam, S. (2006). 'Drugs Cure Depression in Half of Patients'. *The Washington Post*, 23 March 2006, p. A1.
Wear, D. (1998). 'On White Coats and Professional Development: The Formal and the Hidden Curricula'. *Annals of Internal Medicine*, 129(9), pp. 740–42.
Wing, J.K. (1962). 'Institutionalism in Mental Hospitals'. *British Journal of Social Psychology*, 1, pp. 38–51.
World Health Organization (2005). *Mental Health Atlas. Country Profiles*. Geneva: World Health Organization.
—— (2011). *Mental Health Atlas*. Geneva: World Health Organization.
—— (2012). *European Health for All Database*. Available at <http://data.euro.who.int/hfadb/>, accessed 15 June 2012.
Žižek, S. (2009). *Violence*. London: Profile Books.
Zubin, J., and Spring, B. (1977). 'Vulnerability: A New View of Schizophrenia'. *Journal of Abnormal Psychology*, 86(2), pp. 103–2.

Index

Abraham, Karl 57n
aetiology *see* aetiopathogenesis
aetiopathogenesis 13, 18–22, 25, 27, 91, 150–51, 156
Agamben, Giorgio 7, 143–45, 175
alienità 53–55, 57–59, 177, 184, 188
alterità see otherness/other
anti-psychiatry 10, 25, 68–74, 83, 111, 138, 147
antipsychotics 20, 23, 99, 108, 157, 165
  see also drugs; psychopharmacology
Aristotle 49
Artaud, Antonin 68n
authentic/inauthentic existence 53–54, 58–59, 98

Basaglia, Vittorio 127
Battie, William 21, 60
being-in-the-world 30, 41, 52–53, 176
Belloni, Giovanni Battista 13, 15–16, 24, 37, 65
Berg, Jan Hendrik van den 43
Binswanger, Ludwig 10, 14, 18, 25, 29–33, 37, 40, 42, 44, 56, 74–75, 176
biological markers *see* markers, biological
biopolitics 6–7, 9–11, 140–45, 147–49, 157, 160–63, 169, 171, 179–83, 186, 190–92
  affirmative 10–11, 143, 145, 163, 170–71, 179, 181, 183, 190–92
biopower 6, 139, 142–45, 160, 183
biopsychosocial model 18, 151, 159, 162, 164, 168–69
biosecurity 161–63, 169

Bleuler, Eugen 37n
body
  anatomical (*Körper*) 14, 49–50, 61, 112, 127, 141, 148, 185
  economic 110, 186
  institutionalised 36, 60–63, 73
  lived (*Leib*) 36, 48, 49–52, 59–60, 62, 148, 184–86
  social 80, 110, 130, 141, 180, 183–84, 186
bracketing mental illness 106–11, 115, 120, 125, 178, 180, 189
Bukovsky, Vladimir 67

Canguilhem, Georges 73–75, 112, 115–16
Cardiazol 120
Carothers, A. 67
centri di salute mentale (*CSM*) 1, 130, 165–66
Cerletti, Ugo 19
chlorpromazine 20, 155
  see also drugs
Codice Rocco 22–23
coenesthesis 50
colonialism 68, 73
Colorno 4, 11, 17, 96, 127, 138
community
  communitas 171, 181–82, 184, 188, 190
  therapeutic 14, 16, 24, 70–71, 99, 100–2, 120, 127, 184, 186, 190
Cooper, David 10, 69–70, 138, 147
custodialism *see* institutionalism/ custodialism

Dasein 29–30, 41, 43–44, 47, 53, 56, 176
Daseinsanalyse 14–15, 29–33, 36, 41, 42, 111, 189
　see also psychiatry; phenomenological/existentialist
Daumézon, Georges 14, 75
deinstitutionalisation 9, 16, 66, 95–96, 103, 114, 116–18, 126–28, 131, 133, 159, 165–66, 182
Derrida, Jacques 81
Descartes, René 49, 81
diagnosis, psychiatric 19, 21, 37, 54, 70, 82, 88, 98, 105, 114–15, 117, 124, 150–55, 159, 165
Dilthey, Wilhelm 26–28
discipline *see* power, disciplinary; society, disciplinary
drugs 20, 23, 99, 108, 155, 157, 167
　see also psychopharmacology
DSM (*Diagnostic and Statistic Manual*)
　DSM-I 19
　DSM-II 150
　DSM-IV-TR (*Text Revision*) 152–54

ECT (Electro-Convulsive Therapy) 16, 19, 20, 108, 150
edificazione della persona see ontogenesis of the self (*edificazione della persona*)
electroshock *see* ECT
encounter, phenomenological 31, 43–47, 56, 126
Eng, Erling 184–85
Engel, George Libman 18, 162
epoché (phenomenological reduction) 107
ergo-therapy 21, 127
Esposito, Roberto 11, 50, 143–44, 171, 174, 176, 181–84, 188–91
ethopolitics 160–63

existentialism 14, 25, 29, 30, 32, 35, 42, 48, 75–77, 115
Ey, Henry 75

Fanon, Frantz 10, 67–69, 73, 103
Fascism 14, 22
Foucault, Michel 6–7, 25, 60, 71–72, 74–93, 95–97, 111–12, 124–25, 131, 133, 135–44, 146–48, 161–62, 166–67, 171–79, 184, 190
freniatria (phreniatria) 3, 22
Freud, Sigmund 18, 22, 24, 31–32, 57–58, 91

gap (*intervallo*) 36, 55–56, 58, 59, 61, 176, 183–84
gaze 50, 54, 56, 61, 75, 93, 112, 146, 184
Gentile, Giovanni 22
Goffman, Erving 15, 61, 69, 72–73, 87, 105, 122
Gorizia 4, 11, 14, 16, 23, 59, 65–66, 71, 96, 99, 101, 103, 113, 114, 118, 126–27, 129, 137–38
governamentality 141, 149, 160, 163
Gramsci, Antonio 122, 124
Gusdorf, Georges 75

Häfner, Heinz 57–58
Heidegger, Martin 25, 29–32, 53, 76, 176
homo sacer 144–45
hospitalisation, involuntary 1–3, 8, 13, 128–30, 166
Husserl, Edmund 17, 25, 27–28, 30, 49–50, 61, 107, 148, 177

ICD-10 (International Classification of Diseases) 115, 152
immunity (*immunitas*) 50, 171, 181–83, 190
individuality/individual 35n, 48, 86, 140, 169, 172–75, 179, 182, 188–89

Index

institutionalisation 13, 21, 60, 98, 108–9, 172
institutionalism/custodialism 22–24, 37–38, 60
intellectuals 11, 97, 112, 121–26, 178
intersubjectivity 35, 40, 47, 58, 108, 126, 176–77, 179–80, 184–89
intervallo see gap (*intervallo*)

Jaspers, Karl 10, 14, 19, 25–31, 39

Kingsley Hall 70–71, 120, 138
Kraepelin, Emil 19, 152

Lacan, Jacques 75
Lagache, Daniel 75
Laing, Ronald David 10, 25, 69–71, 79, 88, 122, 138
legge 180/1978 (Legge Basaglia) 1–3, 5, 11, 13, 15, 17, 127–32, 138, 164, 167–68, 172, 189
legge 36/1904 3, 22, 97, 107–8, 128, 130
legge stralcio 431/1968 (Legge Mariotti) 22–23, 128–29
lobotomy *see* psychosurgery
Lombroso, Cesare 90–91

Mannheim, Karl 60n–61n
Marco Cavallo 4, 127
Mariotti, Luigi 129
markers, biological 151
Marx, Karl 123
Marxism 60, 76–77n
medicine 22, 54, 61, 73, 82–83, 88, 99, 107, 111–12, 147–48, 151, 160
Merleau-Ponty, Maurice 48, 51, 75
Minkowski, Eugène 36, 44

Nazism 14, 67–68, 144–45
neomanicomialità see reinstitutionalisation

neuroleptics 20
  see also antipsychotics; drugs; psychopharmacology
neurosciences 18, 148
neurosis 57, 60, 71, 91
neurotransmitters 150, 155, 163, 169

objectification 54n, 83, 104, 169, 172, 177
Ongaro Basaglia, Franca 3, 15, 65, 73
ontogenesis of the self (*edificazione della persona*) 42, 48, 52, 57, 61
ospedale psichiatrico giudiziario (OPG) 2, 16, 166
otherness/other (*alterità*) 48, 50–61, 88, 177, 181, 184–85, 188

phenomenology 16–17, 25, 27–29, 39, 77n, 107
phreniatria *see freniatria* (phreniatria)
Pinel, Philippe 71–72, 82–83, 119
Plato 49
population 138–39, 141–42, 160–62, 169–70, 179–80, 186
power
  disciplinary 6–8, 11, 18, 27, 60, 66, 77n, 84–87, 89, 92, 96, 125, 133, 135, 137–42, 148, 161
  sovereign 6–7, 81, 84–86, 125, 137, 140, 142–44, 161, 162, 173, 174
productivity 109, 157
Prozac 155
  see also drugs
psikhushkas 67
psychiatry
  biological (*organicismo*) 21, 23–24, 66
  biological ('first') 8, 10, 13, 15–16, 21–25, 27, 21, 37–40, 46, 54n, 66, 69, 75, 79, 84, 107–8, 111, 115, 117, 132–33, 135, 138, 150, 169, 172

psychiatry, *cont.*
   biological ('second') 5, 149–64, 166
   'biopolitical' 5–7, 9–11, 138, 145–49, 163, 169–70, 171, 191
   'disciplinary' 7–9, 84–85, 87, 89, 92, 96–97, 135, 138, 145, 149, 167, 187
   existentialist *see* psychiatry, phenomenological/existentialist
   institutional 6–10, 13, 16, 31, 37, 39, 46, 66, 68n, 69, 72, 84, 96–97, 101, 104–5, 107–9, 111, 113–14, 115, 118, 124, 131, 132–33, 135, 149, 168–69, 172, 187
   phenomenological/existentialist 14–15, 25–30, 35–40, 45–46, 69, 74–75, 77, 104–5, 107, 175, 184; *see also* Daseinsanalyse
   social 24, 70, 104, 111, 132, 178
psychoanalysis 18, 21–22, 24, 31–32, 45–46, 57–58, 91, 158
psychopathology 14, 19, 26–30, 39, 75
psychopharmacology 155, 157, 161, 164, 166, 191
   cosmetic 161, 164
psychosurgery 3, 13, 20, 98
psychosis 47–48, 52, 57–58
   functional psychoses 19, 151, 159
psychotherapy 21, 24, 44, 147, 188

reductionism, biological 38, 163, 169–70, 172
reinstitutionalisation (*neomanicomialità*) 8, 159, 167

Sartre, Jean Paul 54–56, 59, 73, 123, 126, 131
schizoidia 37, 42

schizophrenia 20n, 28, 69, 70–71, 79, 88, 151, 156–57
servizio psichiatrico di diagnosi e cura (SPDC) 1–2, 131, 164, 166n
shock therapies *see* therapy, shock
society, disciplinary 89, 138, 139–42, 148–49
sovereignty *see* power, sovereign
SSRI (Selective Serotonin Reuptake Inhibitor) 155–57
   see also drugs
stress-vulnerability model 162
subjectivity/subject 27, 32, 35–36, 40, 47–51, 55–56, 60, 115, 132, 140, 164, 169, 171, 172–79, 181, 183–89, 191–92
Szasz, Thomas 10, 69, 73–74, 122, 138, 147

thanatopolitics 6, 10–11, 143–45, 182–83, 190–92
therapy
   convulsive 21, 120; *see also* Cardiazol; ECT; shock therapy
   shock 3, 8, 13, 16, 38, 98, 127
thrownness 53
tricyclics 155
   see also drugs
Trieste 4, 11, 16–17, 65, 96, 101, 110, 118, 120, 127–28, 130, 136, 138
TSO (*Trattamento sanitario obbligatorio*) *see* hospitalisation, involuntary

utopia 10–11, 97, 117–20, 131, 171, 177–78, 181–82, 188–91

Zanetti, Michele 65, 128

ITALIAN MODERNITIES

Edited by
Pierpaolo Antonello and Robert Gordon,
University of Cambridge

The series aims to publish innovative research on the written, material and visual cultures and intellectual history of modern Italy, from the 19th century to the present day. It is open to a wide variety of different approaches and methodologies, disciplines and interdisciplinary fields: from literary criticism and comparative literature to archival history, from cultural studies to material culture, from film and media studies to art history. It is especially interested in work which articulates aspects of Italy's particular, and in many respects, peculiar, interactions with notions of modernity and postmodernity, broadly understood. It also aims to encourage critical dialogue between new developments in scholarship in Italy and in the English-speaking world.

Proposals are welcome for either single-author monographs or edited collections (in English and/or Italian). Please provide a detailed outline, a sample chapter, and a CV. For further information, contact the series editors, Pierpaolo Antonello (paa25@cam.ac.uk) and Robert Gordon (rscg1@cam.ac.uk).

Vol. 1   Olivia Santovetti: *Digression: A Narrative Strategy in the Italian Novel*. 260 pages, 2007.
ISBN 978-3-03910-550-2

Vol. 2   Julie Dashwood and Margherita Ganeri (eds):
The Risorgimento of Federico De Roberto. 339 pages, 2009.
ISBN 978-3-03911-858-8

Vol. 3   Pierluigi Barrotta and Laura Lepschy with Emma Bond (eds):
Freud and Italian Culture. 252 pages, 2009.
ISBN 978-3-03911-847-2

Vol. 4 Pierpaolo Antonello and Florian Mussgnug (eds):
Postmodern Impegno: Ethics and Commitment in Contemporary Italian Culture. 354 pages, 2009.
ISBN 978-3-0343-0125-1

Vol. 5 Florian Mussgnug: *The Eloquence of Ghosts: Giorgio Manganelli and the Afterlife of the Avant-Garde.*
257 pages, 2010.
ISBN 978-3-03911-835-9

Vol. 6 Christopher Rundle: *Publishing Translations in Fascist Italy.*
268 pages, 2010.
ISBN 978-3-03911-831-1

Vol. 7 Jacqueline Andall and Derek Duncan (eds): *National Belongings: Hybridity in Italian Colonial and Postcolonial Cultures.*
251 pages, 2010.
ISBN 978-3-03911-965-3

Vol. 8 Emiliano Perra: *Conflicts of Memory: The Reception of Holocaust Films and TV Programmes in Italy, 1945 to the Present.* 299 pages, 2010.
ISBN 978-3-03911-880-9

Vol. 9 Alan O'Leary: *Tragedia all'italiana: Italian Cinema and Italian Terrorisms, 1970–2010.* 300 pages, 2011.
ISBN 978-3-03911-574-7

Vol. 10 Robert Lumley: *Entering the Frame: Cinema and History in the Films of Yervant Gianikian and Angela Ricci Lucchi.*
228 pages. 2011.
ISBN 978-3-0343-0113-8

Vol. 11 Enrica Maria Ferrara: *Calvino e il teatro: storia di una passione rimossa.* 284 pages, 2011.
ISBN 978-3-0343-0176-3

Vol. 12 Niamh Cullen: *Piero Gobetti's Turin: Modernity, Myth and Memory.* 343 pages, 2011.
ISBN 978-3-0343-0262-3

Vol. 13 Jeffrey T. Schnapp: *Modernitalia*. 338 pages, 2012.
ISBN 978-3-0343-0762-8

Vol. 14 Eleanor Canright Chiari: *Undoing Time: The Cultural Memory of an Italian Prison*. 275 pages, 2012.
ISBN 978-3-0343-0256-2

Vol. 15 Alvise Sforza Tarabochia: *Psychiatry, Subjectivity, Community: Franco Basaglia and Biopolitics*. 226 pages, 2013.
ISBN 978-3-0343-0893-9

www.ingramcontent.com/pod-product-compliance
Ingram Content Group UK Ltd.
Pitfield, Milton Keynes, MK11 3LW, UK
UKHW021845140426
5217IPUK00022B/1597